Nursing care of the patient with burns

# Nursing care of
# the patient with burns

**FLORENCE GREENHOUSE JACOBY, R.N.**

Burn Nurse Clinician,
Strong Memorial Hospital Nursing Service,
The University of Rochester Medical Center,
Rochester, New York

With 17 illustrations, including 2 color plates

**5 5 6 9**

**THE C. V. MOSBY COMPANY**
Saint Louis   1972

Printed in the United States of America

International Standard Book Number 0-8016-2395-2

Library of Congress Catalog Card Number 74-175190

Distributed in Great Britain by Henry Kimpton, London

TO MY HUSBAND

# Preface

When I first became interested in learning more about nursing the burned patient, I searched for a text on the subject written by a nurse. I could not find one. I determined to remedy this situation. This was many years ago. As I researched the field of burn knowledge, I learned the reason why a burn nursing text had not been written by a nurse: the field is extremely complex. Writing a meaningful text on the subject involves many pitfalls.

The material presented here is the result of extensive research of burn literature. Except for personal communications, I have deliberately limited the references to material readily available. I have attended burn teaching seminars throughout the United States and have made many observation visits to hospital facilities caring for burn patients. Most important of all, I have spent many years giving direct nursing care to the burned patient at all stages of care. Today, in my role as a Burn Nurse Clinician, I am involved with improving patient care and helping people discover that nursing the burn patient can be one of the most satisfying and rewarding careers.

Burn care is challenging. It can also be one of the most confusing and frustrating areas for a nurse who does not have some specialized background knowledge in this field. Extensive preparation is not necessary for the nurse who is well grounded in the fundamentals of nursing techniques.

There is no best way or set routine in caring for a burned patient. The only point of burn care that physicians will agree on is that there is still much to be learned. The treatment used depends on the experience of the physician and on the physical facilities and personnel available for giving care. The costs of hospital burn treatment are very high. They can run as high as a thousand dollars for each percent of burn.

In order to work effectively, the nurse should have some knowledge of the fundamental pathologic, physiologic, and psychologic changes that can occur in the burn patient. The nurse must also know some of the specialized techniques and materials used in burn care.

In this book I will present facts that should help a nurse to function efficiently in any setting. There is no mystique in good burn nursing, only a need for understanding. Proper utilization of knowledge will enable a nurse to "think" burn care.

The references listed at the end of each chapter are intended for those interested in in-depth study. *The International Bibliography, Burns,* edited by Dr. Irving Feller, Director of the Burn Center at the University of Michigan, Ann Arbor, and published by the American Burn Research Corp., should be available to all those interested in furthering their knowledge in the burn field.

I am grateful to the many physicians and nurses who guided and encouraged the development of my experience and understanding of the treatment of burns: Dr. Robert McCormack; Dr. Harold Bales; Dr. John Morton; Dr. Lester Cramer; Mrs. Betty Deffenbaugh, R.N.; Mrs. Janet Mance, R.N.; Mrs. Marilyn McClellan, R.N.; Mrs. Kathryn Smith, R.N.; and Mrs. Margaret van der Meer, R.N.

Special mention must be made of Dr. Howard Harrison, whose teaching and help were invaluable.

Personal discussions and correspondence with leaders in the burn field enabled me to develop an overview of burn treatment: Drs. Wesley Alexander, Curtis Artz, Charles Baxter, John Boswick, John Constable, George Crikelair, Irving Feller, Charles Fox, Boyd Haynes, J. Raymond Hinshaw, Duane Larsen, Bruce McMillan, John Moncrief, Carl Moyer, Hiram Polk, Basil Pruitt, Harlan Stone, and Nelson Stone.

I give thanks to Dr. Harold Bales, Mr. George Chernowitz, Mr. Kenneth Elliott, Dr. Howard Harrison, Dr. Earl Parrish, and Dr. Phillip Stoddard for the photographs and illustrations used in the text.

Mrs. Lucretia McClure, librarian, and her staff, of the Edward G. Miner Medical Library, of Strong Memorial Hospital, were most helpful in obtaining the necessary books and reference materials.

I am most grateful to Mr. Moses Capell, close friend and advisor.

To my sons Stuart, Richard, and Robert, a special thanks is due for their cooperation and understanding.

Finally, I am eternally grateful to my husband, Marvin, who assisted in the preparation of the manuscript and whose encouragement kept my spirits from faltering.

Florence Greenhouse Jacoby

# Contents

# CHAPTER 1

# Incidence of burns, provisions for care, and goals

## EXTENT OF LOSSES

The American Insurance Association's estimate of fire losses in the United States during 1969 was $1,952,000,000. The National Safety Council reports 115,000 accidental deaths from all causes in 1969. Fires, burns, and other injuries associated with the burning process accounted for 7,100 deaths in that year.

In 1967 the National Safety Council and the National Center for Health Statistics reported 7,423 deaths caused by fire and explosion of combustible materials. The National Center for Health Statistics also listed 992 deaths caused by electric current; 376 deaths caused by hot substances, corrosive materials, and steam; and 42 deaths caused by explosion of pressure vessels. Since all these deaths usually involved burn injury of some type, these figures should be grouped together, making the total 8,833 deaths.

For the years 1965 to 1967, the National Center for Health Statistics reported an annual average of 2,230,000 burn injuries. Of these 682,000 occurred at work, 1,291,000 occurred at home, and 34,600 are classified as "other." Over 1,333,000 victims of burn injury received medical attention but did not need to restrict their activity as a result. Some 599,000 burn victims who were medically attended had activity-restricting injuries; of these, 359,000 were serious enough to confine the patient to bed.

## NEED FOR HOSPITALIZATION

In 1965, 91,000 burn patients were admitted for in-hospital care. The average stay in the hospital was 14.8 days. This figure, for the most part, would apply to those patients not needing grafting procedures. For cases involving grafting, 1 to 3 months is a more realistic figure. Various complications can prolong the initial hospitalization period to 6 months or more.

## DISTRIBUTION OF BURN INJURY

Of the 2,233,000 people who suffered burn injuries each year from 1965 through 1967, the number of males injured was 1,297,000 and the number of females, 936,000. The burn injuries during this same period, according to geographic distribution, were:

| | |
|---|---|
| North East | 496,000 |
| North Central | 674,000 |
| South | 770,000 |
| West | 293,000 |

The hospital admissions by age groups are divided as follows:

| | |
|---|---|
| Under age 15 | 33,000 |
| 15 to 44 | 34,000 |
| 45 to 64 | 18,000 |
| Over 65 | 6,000 |

The Shriner's Burn Institute of Galveston, Texas, has a thirty-bed burn unit for the treatment of children. Of 854 burned children aged 1 month to 15 years treated during a 3-year period, 455 were boys and 399 were girls. Until age 9, the ratio of boys to girls was one to one. After age 9, the burn-injured boys outnumbered the girls three to one.

## CAUSES OF BURN INJURY

Gasoline and other volatile liquids caused 80% of the burn injuries of the boys at Galveston. Open gas space heaters caused 80% of the burns in young girls. Hot liquids, such as bath water or spilled hot cooking liquids, accounted for 15% of the burn injuries of all children. Flaming clothing, which was involved in 56% of the burn injuries, increases the severity of the burn injury. The campaign for the use of flame-retardent clothing for all age groups must be intensified. The federal government is studying the matter.

Three fourths of the burn injuries of children could have been prevented.

With the ever-expanding population, especially in big cities, the advent of the huge airliners, and the possibility of nuclear explosions, hospitals must be prepared to treat increasing numbers of burn victims.

## PROVISION FOR BURN CARE

As of 1969, special facilities for burn care were available for only 9% of the burn victims requiring hospital admission.

A burn referral center can be any hospital that has the necessary personnel and equipment to provide the multidisciplinary approach needed for burn care. A burn unit can be a separate facility, such as the Shriner's Burn Institutes in Galveston, Boston, and Cincinnati, or it can be a separate floor in a hospital. Some hospitals have a few rooms reserved for burn care. Ideally, a burn unit has its own operating and dressing rooms. A facility for hydrotherapy and physiotherapy should also be readily available.

The number of specialized burn units is increasing each year. The majority of burn victims, though, are still being treated in general hospitals having no specialized burn unit. This book is intended as a guide to help organize burn care in hospitals of this type.

## ORGANIZATION OF BURN CARE

The key to successful burn care in a medical facility not having a burn unit is the organization of a burn service. This would imply that the physicians responsible for administering hospital policies have set up treatment guides relating to the admission and care of the burned patient. These policies should be available in the form of written guides available to all personnel involved in administering burn care (see Chapters 5 and 14). These procedure manuals should be the type to lend themselves easily to revision (loose leaf).

In an organized burn unit, an orientation period for new employees familiarizes them with the theory and practice of burn work. In a general hospital, supervisory personnel and in-service instructors would have to take the responsibility of acquainting staff members with the procedures and policies of burn care. If a procedure manual is available to the staff, implementation of care is greatly facilitated.

Physicians can play a major role in training nurses in burn care techniques. Attendance of nurses and therapists at burn teaching seminars given at burn unit centers, such as the University Hospital, Ann Arbor, Michigan, and the Sumner Koch Burn Unit at the Cook County Hospital, Chicago, Illinois, is most helpful.

Most important of all is the fact that the physicians playing major roles today in the burn field recognize the importance of the role that nurses and paramedical personnel can play in providing care for the burned patient. These physicians need only to be asked to provide guidance and direction for such programs.

Turnover of personnel at staff levels would tend to focus attention on the importance of the role of the clinician or burn nurse specialist to provide for continuity of care. The nurse clinician, working closely with the physician, would help coordinate the burn program and serve as a consultant for teaching the theory and practice of burn care.

Most institutions treating large numbers of burn victims have established care patterns. Each feels that its particular method of treatment is the most effective. Yet there is a tremendous variance of treatment from one institution to another. When nurses are presented with the basic information, they will understand why the various treatment methods can vary so and yet be comparatively equally effective.

## BURN CARE OBJECTIVES

While physical facilities and the experience of personnel involved in burn care may vary greatly, the basic goals of care do not. The objectives of all burn care and treatment can be stated as follows:
1. Prevention and treatment of shock
2. Alleviation of pain
3. Control of bacterial growth on the burn wound and within the body
4. Conversion of the open wound to a closed wound
5. Preservation of body function and appearance
6. Healing within a minimal period of time
7. Preservation of the mental and emotional equilibrium of the patient

## PHASES OF BURN CARE

The course of burn care can be divided into three phases. The first is commonly referred to as the acute phase. Other terms also used are emergent phase, metabolic phase, or resuscitative phase. The major problems during this period are caused by the injured vasculature, with resulting increased permeability. The fluid and electrolyte balances are often difficult to control.

A period of reabsorption takes place after approximately 48 hours or longer, depending on the general physical condition of the patient, the severity of the burn injury, and the kind and amount of fluids given.

When the excess fluid in the body is sequestered and then excreted by the kidneys, diuresis is said to occur. This can be a gradual process or a more dramatic occurrence. The patient who has been voiding in 50- to 100-ml. quantities may void 1,000 ml. or more.

The second phase of burn care is referred to as the wound or management phase. This can last for only a matter of a few weeks or for many months. Infection in the burn wounds and some form of pneumonia invariably appear early in this period. The goals during this period are:
1. Wound cleansing
2. Preparation for grafting, if needed

3. Prevention and minimizing of infection
4. Closure of burn wounds, with preservation of body function
5. Meeting the nutritional and psychologic needs of the patient

For most major burns requiring grafting, the goal is to do the first autograft within 3 weeks and to discharge the patient from the hospital within 3 months.

The third phase of burn care is the rehabilitative phase. This period may start in the hospital as the burn wounds are being closed. Psychologic support is given the patient to help with the eventual adjustment to everyday living. Social workers can help with plans.

The nature of the burn wound is such that a period of time must elapse to allow the scar tissue of the wound to mature. Some scars regress and do not need further work. Other wound conditions, such as excess hypertrophy of scar tissue or contractures, require corrective surgery during the years following the initial burn injury. This period may last for many years, or until the physician and the patient feel that the maximum amount of function and appearance are restored.

Burn care needs to be definitive and aggressive in order to sustain the patient and to secure healing in the minimum amount of time.

## THE BURN TEAM

No one person can meet all the needs of the severely burned patient. The physician in charge may need the help of other physicians, plastic surgeons, orthopedists, physiatrists, and psychiatrists. Other members of the burn team include nurses, physical therapists, occupational therapists, recreational therapists, nutritionists, teachers, social workers, family, friends, and clergy.

## REFERENCES

National Center for Health Statistics, Series 13, No. 6, May, 1970.

National Safety Council: Condensed facts, July, 1970.

Personal communications with Drs. C. Artz, H. Bales, C. Baxter, J. Boswick, I. Feller, D. Larson, R. McCormack, B. MacMillan, J. Moncrief, J. Morton, B. Pruitt, and C. Rob.

Stone, N. H., and Boswick, J. A.: Profiles of burn management, Miami, 1969, Industrial Medicine Publishing Co.

# CHAPTER 2

# Anatomy of the skin
# and
# burn wound classification

The skin is composed of two layers: the outer layer is called the epidermis, the inner layer, either dermis or corium. The epidermis consists of stratified squamous epithelial tissue, the dermis of fibrous connective tissue. Underlying the dermis is the loose subcutaneous tissue, which is made up of areolar, and in some cases adipose, tissue. This overlays the subcutaneous fat pad.

The terms "thick skin" and "thin skin" are frequently used. In the areas of thick skin—the palms of the hands and the soles of the feet—the epidermis has five layers. In the areas of thin skin—all other body surfaces—the epidermis has only four layers.

## EPIDERMIS

The five epidermal layers are, from the surface inward: stratum corneum, stratum lucidum (this layer is missing in "thin skin"), stratum granulosum, stratum spinosum, and stratum germinativum (this layer abuts on the dermis).

The stratum corneum is composed of keratin fibers surrounded by a lipid monolayer. Since lipids are water repellant, this layer acts as the vapor barrier for the body. When large areas of the stratum corneum are damaged, as in a burn (even one of a very superficial type), extensive fluid loss occurs, adding greatly to the fluids that must be replaced. This loss is of electrolyte-free water and must be replaced as such.

The innermost layer, the stratum germinativum, is also of great importance. This layer constantly produces new cells that move toward the surface and so renew the other epidermal layers. It is the presence of this layer that determines whether or not a burned area will require grafting. If all vestiges of it are destroyed, regeneration cannot take place.

## DERMIS OR CORIUM

The dermis, or corium, serves as a supporting and nutritional bed for the epidermis. The dermis is composed of two layers. The outermost layer (that next to the epidermis) is called the papillary layer; the innermost layer is called the reticular layer. The predominant fiber in the dermis is collagen. Scattered through the collagen are connective tissue cells (the mast cells) performing the functions of secretion, phagocytosis (the histiocytes), and repair (the fibroblasts). In a burn injury, the mast cells pour out increased amounts of histamine.

## EPIDERMAL APPENDAGES

The epidermal appendages are found in the dermis. They include the hair follicles, the sebaceous glands, and the sweat glands. When a burn destroys the epidermal layer, the epithelial cells of the external sheaths of the hair follicles and sebaceous and sweat glands can grow out to form new epithelium.

The hair follicles may harbor the bacteria that are normally part of the flora of the skin. Burn trauma upsets the normal functioning of the skin's protective mechanisms. Sebaceous glands secrete sebum, which contains fatty acids, including oleic acid. In addition to lubricating the skin, sebum can destroy streptococci and some strains of staphylococci. In burn trauma much serum is lost from damaged capillaries. This serum provides rich nutritional support for bacterial growth. Bacteria can multiply very rapidly on the surface of a burn wound moistened by this serous exudate. Bacteria do not multiply as fast when conditions are dry, so colonization can be slowed on the burn wound surface if the involved areas are kept as free of serous exudate as possible. Even under the best conditions these wounds can develop burn wound sepsis.

These are some of the basic facts that must be considered when evaluating the efficacy of the various methods employed in the local care of the burn wound. Unless there is an effective antimicrobial agent used, wound surfaces should be kept as dry as possible. Exposure therapy and wet or dry dressings (see Chapter 4) must be properly handled in order to keep the burn wound free of septic involvement and to prepare it promptly for grafting.

A fairly reliable test to determine the depth of burn injury is the hair test. If hair can be easily pulled out, a full-thickness injury is usually present.

## SUBCUTANEOUS TISSUE (SUBCUTANEOUS FASCIA)

The skin rests on subcutaneous tissue that is areolar and adipose in character. Collagen fibers extending from the dermis anchor the skin to this subcutaneous layer. These collagen fibers play an important role in the treatment of the burn wound. They anchor the burn slough or eschar firmly in place, making removal of the slough and eschar difficult. The fibers are dissolved by the lytic enzymes released by the bacteria inhabiting an infected burn wound. The eschar of such burns separates at an earlier time than that from a clean wound.

## MELANIN

The skin is pigmented by a substance called melanin, which occurs as an inclusion in the cytoplasm of the skin. Cells containing melanin are found in the epidermis and dermis. The amount of melanin in the skin determines a person's color. Exposure to ultraviolet light increases the amount of melanin. Dark-haired people tan more easily than people with light hair. In some cases the melanin is produced in patches and freckles result. It is thought that the melanin in the skin affords protection against sunlight. The melanocyte does not regenerate readily; in deep burns the skin color may not return.

## NERVE FIBERS

The nerve fibers in the skin come from a nerve plexus deep in the dermis. Naked nerve endings between the layers of the stratum germinativum receive pain sensation. The pin prick test is often used to ascertain the depth of burn injury, but this is not a particularly reliable test for initial evaluation.

The sensation of touch is provided by Meissner's corpuscles, which are located just below the epidermis. The corpuscles of Vater-Pacini (for pressure) and of Ruffini (for heat) and Krause's end-bulbs (for cold) are all located in the dermis and subcutaneous fascia. A deeply burned patient, therefore, rarely complains of pain, while a patient with partial-thickness burns does. Sensory function returns to the skin about 2 months after grafting, but the nerve regeneration process may continue for many years.

## BLOOD SUPPLY

The largest skin arteries are found in the rete cutaneum, a flat network in the subcutaneous tissue just beneath the dermis. Branches of this network pass inward to supply the superficial portions of the subcutaneous tissue, while outward branches supply the skin. When these branches reach the reticular layer of the dermis, they form a second flat network called the rete subpapillare. The capillary beds of the skin are most abundant in the area of the epidermal appendages.

Arterioles from the rete subpapillare supply tissue fluid to the basal cell layer of the epidermis. The epidermis itself has no blood vessels; the pink color of the skin comes from the subpapillary plexi of the skin, generally described as venous plexi. They consist of capillaries and small venules.

The extensive papillary and subpapillary plexi of the skin account for the marked color changes seen in thermal injury. Sunburn will cause these vessels to dilate, thus producing a marked reddening. In severe burns, the coagulation of the blood vessels can cause the affected area to lose all redness and appear almost white at first.

Plasma leaking from the heat-changed blood vessels can cause edema and blistering. In thick skin (on the palms of the hands and on the soles of the feet) blisters may result from intraepithelial accumulations of plasma. In thin skin, blisters result from plasma accumulations between the epidermis and the dermis.

## LYMPH

The lymphatic vessels, which are arranged in superficial and in deep networks, are particularly numerous in the skin. In burn injury, the lymphatic vessels become permeable and then cannot fulfill their normal drainage function. This contributes to the problem of edema. Because of their thin walls the lymphatics are the first circulatory vessels to be closed by the edema of the burn. At times these must be decompressed by splitting the burned skin surgically (escharotomy or fasciotomy).

## BURN WOUND CLASSIFICATION

Various forms of classification are used to describe the severity of a burn injury. The terms "first," "second," "third," and sometimes "fourth-degree" burn are commonly used. This classification is based on the surface appearance of the burn wound.

The trend today is toward the use of the terms "partial thickness," "deep dermal," and "full thickness" in describing burn wounds. The term "partial thickness" is used to describe a wound that has the ability to heal without grafting. The wound can resurface itself from the stratum germinativum of the epidermis. The deepest epithelial cells capable of regeneration are present in the sheaths of the epidermal appendages, deep in the dermis and subcutaneous tissue.

A deep dermal burn is a partial-thickness wound that frequently has the gross appearance of a third-degree, or full-thickness, burn. It can also heal without grafting. However, infection, mechanical trauma, or obliteration of the blood supply to the affected part can destroy the deep epithelial cells and convert a partial-thickness deep dermal burn wound to a full-thickness wound.

In a full-thickness burn wound all the epithelializing elements are destroyed, both in the epidermis and in the epidermal appendages. This type of wound must be grafted with autografts in order to be closed properly.

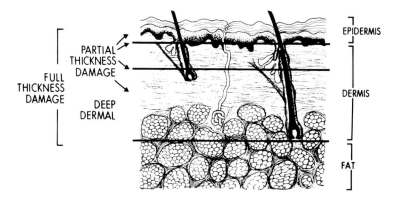

Fig. 2-1. Diagram of skin showing depth of burn. (Courtesy Dr. H. Harrison.)

First-degree, partial-thickness burns involve the epidermal layers. This type of injury can result from moderate to prolonged exposure to the burning rays of the sun, very brief exposure to heat (flash burns), splashes from hot liquids (6- to 10-second exposure to hot liquids produces full-thickness burns), and high-intensity, short-duration explosions. The areas affected appear red or pink. Pain and slight edema are present, but they subside rather quickly. The epidermis peels in 3 to 6 days. Itching and redness may persist for a week or so. There is no scarring.

Second-degree, partial-thickness burns involve the epidermis and the dermis. They are caused by exposure to intense flash heat, immersion or

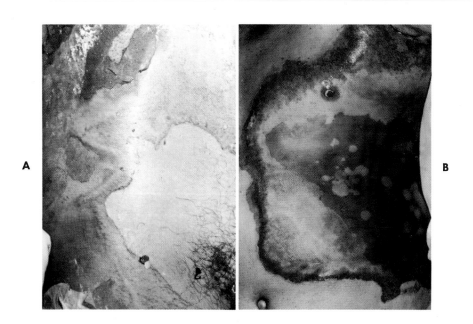

**Plate 1. A,** Partial-thickness gasoline flash burn. White areas are unburned skin. Brown areas are partial-thickness wounds, discolored by gasoline fumes. Dark pink areas are deep partial-thickness wounds that might convert to full-thickness wounds. **B,** Full-thickness contact burn. The complete spectrum of full-thickness wound coloration is demonstrated, ranging from deep cherry-red through white, tan, dark brown, and black. (**A,** Courtesy Dr. H. Bales; **B,** courtesy Dr. P. Stoddard.)

contact with hot liquids, or contact with hot objects. These wounds are further classified into superficial and deep dermal partial-thickness types.

The superficial partial-thickness burn wound appears mottled pink or red. There frequently is blistering and some subcutaneous edema. The wound is usually moist and sensitive. This type of wound can heal in 10 to 14 days with no scarring if it does not become infected or traumatized.

In the deep dermal partial-thickness burn wound much of the dermis and possibly the subcutaneous fat tissue are involved. Some epidermal appendages must be intact in order for these wounds to heal spontaneously. These wounds can vary greatly in appearance. They can be mottled, with white areas predominating over red, or they can be dull white, tan, or cherry red in color. Very often, dark streaks of coagulated capillaries can be seen. The wound can be blistered and moist looking or dry. It may or may not be sensitive to the touch. If hair follicles are present, the hair does not pull out. Burn wounds of this type may take several months to heal. The epithelium produced is very thin. Blistering and tissue breakdown occur very easily. Some deep dermal partial-thickness burns are therefore excised and autografted to provide a more durable coverage and better function. It is now felt that in the period before the development of effective topical antimicrobial therapy, many deep dermal burns were converted from partial thickness to full-thickness wounds by infection.

Third-degree, full-thickness burn wounds have no remaining viable epithelial cells. These wounds can be white, tan, brown, black, or deep cherry red in color. The surface may be wet or dry, is sometimes leathery (the result of surface dehydration), and may have a sunken look. This leathery covering is called eschar. Black networks of coagulated capillaries may be seen. These wounds are usually anesthetic. Wounds of this type, larger than a fifty-cent piece, need to be grafted in order to heal properly.

Fourth-degree, full-thickness burn injuries may involve the subcutaneous fat, fascia, muscle, and bone. The wound usually appears blackened and depressed. When the burn injury includes the bone, it is dull and dry. In order to achieve a granulating surface on which a skin graft can be applied, multiple perforations reaching into the marrow cavity may be made in the bone. This process is called fenestration. Granulating buds appear from these perforations and then coalesce to form a firm bed that will accept a graft.

Autografting with split-thickness skin grafts for coverage of full-thickness burn wounds is started as soon as the patient's condition is stable, skin is available, and the recipient beds are ready.

**REFERENCES**

Anthony, C. P.: Textbook of anatomy and physiology, ed. 7, St. Louis, 1967, The C. V. Mosby Co.

Ham, A. W., and Leeson, T. H.: Histology, ed. 6, Philadelphia, 1969, J. B. Lippincott Co.

Rothman, S.: Physiology and biochemistry of the skin, Chicago, 1954, University of Chicago Press.

Sevitt, S.: Burns—pathology and therapeutic applications, London, 1957, Butterworth & Co. (Publishers) Ltd.

# CHAPTER 3

# Systemic changes caused by burn injury

Burn wounds can result from many causes. Flame, steam, hot liquids, or hot objects can cause thermal burns. Electricity, acids, alkalis and other chemicals, poison gases, x-ray or atomic radiation, and ultraviolet light can cause changes in tissue similar to those seen in thermal burns. In addition to the visible injury manifestated by changes in the appearance of the skin, there are alterations in the vascular system that can cause reduced or altered tissue perfusion, thus disrupting many other systems of the body.

The degree of burn injury is determined by the temperature of the heat source and the length of exposure to it. The severity of the injury depends on the size of the area burned, the depth and location of the burn, the age of the victim, the presence of concomitant illness or injury, and the prior psychologic status of the victim. It is most important to know the circumstances in which the burn injury occurred. Burns occurring in enclosed areas can cause severe respiratory damage. Prolonged contact with objects of relatively low temperature can cause more tissue damage than flash or brief scald wounds. Electrical, radiation, and chemical burns can cause systemic and tissue damage that is far greater than appearance would indicate.

Some people appear to be relatively burn resistant; others have serious problems with what appears to be superficial injury. There appear to be physical, biochemical, and genetic differences among people that affect the outcome of burn injury.

In a burn injury, the protein of the cells comprising the skin tissue is denatured and the enzymes inactivated. The tissue becomes coagulated, desiccated, or carbonized, according to the temperature and length of time

**13**

of exposure to the heat source (just as the white of an egg will change with time and intensity of heat exposure). In any case, even with mild heat, the normal metabolic activity of the cell is disrupted. These changes begin to occur at approximately 42° C. or 107.6° F.

The water vapor barrier for the body is in the stratum corneum, the outermost layer of the epidermis. A very extensive superficial burn may heal in a matter of a few days, but a person can have severe systemic reactions from fluid losses caused by water vaporization from affected skin. In deep burns, fluid is lost until the involved areas heal or are grafted. This continuing fluid loss contributes to the problems of care for the burned patient. Measurements have shown that a severely burned patient can lose as much as 10 liters of fluid a day through apparently dry eschar. This must be considered when calculating for the replacement of fluid losses.

Changes resulting from heat in the intercellular cement, which binds the epidermis to the dermis, causes the epidermis to loosen. The epidermis can then be peeled off readily, or blisters may form between the skin layers.

## CHANGES IN THE CIRCULATORY SYSTEM

The first effect of thermal injury is blanching, which results from contraction of the skin capillaries. If the superficial dermis is coagulated at the same time, the burn wound appears white. Later, the wound reddens as the arterioles and capillaries dilate.

Edema is one of the most characteristic features of a burn wound. When the fluid loss from the capillaries exceeds the rate of fluid return, the tissue fluid is thereby increased and edema develops. This fluid accumulation may appear subcutaneously in the form of blisters. It also causes the characteristic swelling and thickening of the tissue under the burn. In severe cases the fluid may pool deep within the body, away from the burned area.

The permeable capillary walls allow the fluid portion of the blood to escape, so the cellular elements of the blood become more and more concentrated. As a result of this hemoconcentration the hematocrit rises and blood flow becomes sluggish and difficult. This sluggish blood flow may severely compromise tissue nutrition. True thrombi are sometimes seen, but in many cases they are not.

Stasis may have a rapid or delayed onset, but it is an important consideration. If it does develop, the area affected will die. In extensive burns, a large volume of red cells may be trapped in the engorged capillaries and be lost to the body. This, along with red cell lysis, contributes to the anemia that sometimes occurs with burns. Capillary stasis may also prolong edema.

The tissue fluid is physiologically isolated from the capillary bed from which it originated, and that area is lost for fluid resorption.

Circulatory changes caused by the burn injury can cause marked changes in the appearance of the burn wound. These changes can be progressive. Aside from superficial burns, it is very difficult to ascertain the exact nature of burn wounds when first seen. Thrombi developing in the blood vessels, as a result of capillary stasis or heat-changed red blood cells, can cause ischemia and eventually necrosis of the affected part. Capillaries coagulated by heat are seen as dark streaks. The entire capillary plexus, known as a burn angiogram, can very often be seen in an extensive burn. The brownish discoloration of superficial healed burns results from broken-down red blood cells escaping from the vascular system by diapedesis.

Red blood cell destruction can occur immediately in the burned area, or it can be gradual, as partially hemolyzed cells decompose. Hematocrit may be high at first because of fluid volume losses from the intravascular spaces. If the burn injury is extensive or if there is bleeding from other sources, anemia may manifest itself when the fluid volume is restored.

A leukocytosis during the very early phase of burn care may be caused by the decreased fluid volume, resulting in a high white blood cell concentration. Initial tissue damage can affect the neutrophils. The extent of damage depends on the severity of the injury. Leukocytosis manifested after the first week is usually symptomatic of gram-positive infection. Leukopenia may indicate a gram-negative infection.

Body fluids account for 50%, plus or minus 15%, of the weight of the average person. Alterations in the quantity or chemical composition of these fluids disrupt the homeostasis of the body. Homeostasis is the maintenance of the constancy of the internal medium, which is comprised of blood, interstitial tissue fluid, and intracellular fluid. In burn injuries, the homeostasis of the body is disrupted; therefore, all the systems of the body can be affected.

The fluid of the human body is of two types: intracellular and extracellular. Intracellular fluid is found inside each individual cell. Extracellular fluid is found in the intravascular system as plasma and in the tissue spaces as interstitial fluid. These two body fluids are therefore seen to occupy three body compartments: intravascular space, tissue space, and cells.

In an adult, intracellular fluid constitutes approximately 50% of the body weight, interstitial fluid, 15% to 25%, and plasma, 5%. These proportions vary somewhat according to the size and age of the individual. In burn injury, marked systemic changes can occur because of fluid shifts caused by heat changes in the walls of the intravascular system and the destruction of cells. This shift of fluids involves both physical and chemical changes. The physical change derives from a shift in the actual amount of fluid in the various compartments, either increasing or decreasing from normal. The chemical change derives from the change in the electrolyte and chemical content of the various body fluids when they move from one compartment to another.

Plasma and interstitial fluid are chemically similar. The interstitial fluid is composed of those blood components that are capable of passing through capillary walls. The colloid content of normal interstitial fluid is therefore somewhat less than that of blood plasma, because the colloid particles are fairly large and cannot diffuse through the capillary walls. In burn injury, the weakened capillary walls allow colloids to escape readily from the intravascular space into the interstitial spaces. Therefore, there is a loss of the colloid osmotic pressure difference between the capillary plasma and the tissue fluid exudate, and edema develops.

The pumping action of the heart normally creates a hydrostatic pressure in the circulatory system. This pressure drives fluid through the endothelium of the capillary walls, thus producing tissue fluid. The arterial ends of the capillaries are the main source of the body tissue fluid. The movement of this tissue fluid in and out of the capillaries depends on whether the hydrostatic pressure within the capillaries is greater or less than the difference in osmotic pressure between the blood and the tissue fluid. The rate of formation of edema in a burn victim depends on the difference between the capillary hydrostatic pressure and the tissue fluid pressure (bearing in mind that colloid osmotic pressure within the capillary has been lost as a result of capillary permeability, with resultant loss of colloid to the tissue fluid) and on the volume of blood flow through the affected capillaries.

The entire circulatory system of the body is upset by thermal injury. Normally, intravascular fluid containing some protein (colloid) leaves the arterial end of the capillary, enters the interstitial space, and is reabsorbed into the circulatory system by lymphatic drainage and through the venous end of the capillaries. This process depends on:

1. The arterial end of the capillary having greater hydrostatic pressure than the venous end
2. Colloid osmotic pressure of the capillary plasma being greater than that of the tissue fluid
3. The relative impermeability of the capillary endothelium

In a burn injury the capillary endothelium becomes permeable. Plasma escapes from the intravascular space into the interstitial spaces, a process known as sieving. The exact mechanisms involved are not known. The process continues for varying periods of time, usually 36 to 48 hours following the injury. The colloid osmotic pressure difference between the capillary plasma and the interstitial fluid is thereby diminished. The lymphatics cannot handle the fluid load, and edema results. Edema can even occur in areas not burned. In severe burn injuries considerable edema may not be visible but may occur deep within the body.

Capillary permeability can occur immediately following burn injury or at a later period. The delayed effect is usually found in the deep subcutaneous capillaries, although it can also occur in superficial ones. Why it stops is almost as much a mystery as why it starts. No therapeutic substances are known that will reestablish the integrity of the capillary wall once it has been impaired.

The body tries to compensate for the loss of plasma volume by the general constriction of blood vessels. The arterial blood pressure and circulating volume may at first be in the normal range, but if fluid losses are not replaced, hypovolemia occurs within a few hours, depending on the extent of the burn. The body has several natural ways by which it holds arterial pressure up in the face of loss of plasma volume. It can withdraw fluid from undamaged parts of the extracellular space. Blood vessels in the splanchnic area and in the skin can contract, thereby increasing the peripheral resistance, so that blood pressure is maintained and vital organs receive an adequate blood supply.

The burned patient is usually thirsty. He is, however, frequently nauseated and unable to keep down oral fluids. Therefore, oral fluids usually are not offered until normal intestinal peristalsis is present. If a burn is large and the fluid losses are not replaced aggressively by intravenous therapy, splanchnic constriction can lead to gastric dilatation and paralytic ileus. Oral fluids can be given in minor or moderate burn injuries, but in major burns there is danger of aspiration. Well-treated burn patients invariably show a weight gain of about 10% during initial treatment.

The reduction of the circulating blood volume can result in a decrease in cardiac output and inadequate tissue perfusion. The resultant tissue hypoxia causes a cellular shift from an aerobic metabolism to an anaerobic metabolism. Acidosis followed by structural damage and irreversible burn shock can result.

Whole blood contains cells and fluid. There are three main types of cells in the blood: leukocytes, or white corpuscles; erythrocytes, or red corpuscles; and thrombocytes, or platelets. The fluid portion of the blood is called plasma and contains in solution more than 100 different substances, of which some are crystalloid (electrolyte) and some are colloid in nature. Examples of crystalloids or electrolytes are sodium chloride, potassium chloride, and sodium bicarbonate. Examples of colloids are albumin and the globulins.

One of the functions of the blood is to maintain the proper acid-base balance of the body which is frequently disrupted in burn injury. Acid-base balance refers to the maintenance of homeostasis of the hydrogen ion concentration of the body fluids. The symbol pH is used to indicate the state of acidity or alkalinity of the body fluids. Normal body solutions have a pH of 7.4, which represents slight alkalinity. The normal pH of the body is maintained by the respiratory system (which expels carbon dioxide), by the kidneys (which excrete acids and bases), and by chemical buffers in the body fluids.

The buffering mechanism of the burned patient is upset by the fluid shift within the body compartments. The concentration of the sodium, potassium, bicarbonate, and chloride ions and their imbalance caused by the fluid shifts need to be carefully monitored. Direct irritation of the respiratory system, or by hyperventilation, plus reduced effectiveness of the renal tubular function, may result from the burn trauma and contribute to the disruption of the acid-base balance. Therefore, careful periodic monitoring of the serum electrolytes, arterial blood gases, urine volume, and urine electrolytes is needed as a basis for rational fluid therapy.

Extracellular fluid is different chemically from intracellular fluid. Sodium is the main positively-charged ion (cation) of extracellular fluid; potassium is the main cation of the intracellular fluid. Serum potassium levels may rise initially because of potassium release from damaged cells. In severely burned patients, cardiac failure can result from high potassium levels. Potassium is one of the myriad substances excreted by the kidneys. When the patient begins diuresis, significant amounts of potassium are lost. The serum potassium level also needs to be checked periodically, and additional potassium may be required.

Free water and electrolyte fluids need to be given to replace losses during the acute phase of burn therapy. However, excessive water intake can reduce extracellular osmolality, shift into the cells, and cause swelling and the death of these cells. This condition is known as water intoxication.

The plasma sodium level initially can be normal or moderately low, while the chloride is normal or slightly elevated. Sodium and chloride ion levels can rise quite rapidly as burn edema is reabsorbed. Administration of electrolyte fluids needs to be adjusted to these changes by close monitoring of serum electrolytes and urinary losses during the reabsorption phase.

The blood urea level may rise after burn injury if excessive catabolism of proteins occurs or if the injured tissues release large amounts of nitrogen in the face of oliguria.

The blood glucose level has sometimes been seen to be elevated after burn injury. This is most often the result of the dextrose in water solution used in therapy. Lactic acid frequently accumulates during the early post-injury stages. This happens when cells become hypoxic from the loss of circulating blood volume and the lack of tissue perfusion. When this happens, not enough oxygen is present in the cells to convert the glucose to energy. The increased lactic acid level and the loss of electrolytes and water cause a decrease in the alkaline reserves of the body. If vigorous and adequate fluid resuscitation is implemented, the lactic acid level returns to normal, unless primary pulmonary problems exist.

Protein losses can be extensive in burn injury. However, the plasma levels can remain in the normal range as long as adequate nutrition is maintained. Total nitrogen losses occur through the kidneys as well as through the burn wound exudate. Low protein intake and the tendency toward catabolism contribute to the significant negative nitrogen balance frequently seen. Healing can take place in the face of negative nitrogen balance and is surprisingly fast. But if the patient's nutritional status deteriorates, wound healing slows. The debilitated patient may succumb to other complications. Even the most energetic oral nutritional program may not be sufficient to overcome the negative nitrogen balance; intravenous hyperalimentation may be needed from time to time to help bolster the patient's condition.

## CHANGES IN THE RESPIRATORY SYSTEM

The respiratory changes associated with burn injury occur as a result of various factors. These include:

1. Irritation of respiratory tissues caused by inhalation of the products of burning materials (including soot particles and/or gases from the burning materials)
2. The swelling or breakdown of tissue from exposure to irritants or heat
3. Inadequate circulation through the lungs, with resulting hypoxemia
4. Cardiopulmonary pathology prior to injury, such as chronic bronchitis, emphysema, or congestive heart failure
5. Bacterial invasion of the respiratory tract from the environment, the burn wound, or a tracheostomy

Knowledge of the circumstances of the burn injury is helpful in planning for care. Was the patient in an enclosed space? What was the nature of the burning materials? Respiratory symptoms occur at varying times: some immediately, others within a matter of hours, others after a week or more.

Initial physical examination may reveal singed nasal hairs and reddened or darkened pharynx. Bronchoscopic or vocal cord examination may be needed to determine the extent of injury. Initial x-ray findings are very often inconclusive. Treatment regimes are based on relief of symptoms and physical findings, and many of the problems can be anticipated.

Pain and fear contribute to the hyperventilation seen initially in burn victims. Initial restlessness may result from cerebral anoxia, pain, or fear. Exposure to carbon monoxide gas may produce a cherry red color in the lips and skin that masks cyanosis. Humidified oxygen, delivered by a fine-mist nebulizer, immediately on admission when respiratory damage is suspected is essential for the reversal of carbon monoxide inhalation and is generally very helpful. Masks that do not touch the face are available for use with facial burns (see Fig. 6-1).

Irritation and heat changes in the respiratory tract tissues can lead to dyspnea, stridor, and copious mucous secretions. Airway occlusion may result from bronchospasm or laryngospasm, bronchial or laryngeal edema, edema of the peritracheal tissue, and plugs of mucus or tissue slough. Atelectasis can occur very easily.

One should keep in mind that severe respiratory tract damage can occur without extensive body burns if the patient was exposed to the smoke and gaseous products of burning or to steam. On the other hand, patients suffering facial or extensive body burns caused by immersion or contact with a heat source can also develop respiratory complications.

When facial and body burns are present, fluid losses and tissue changes producing edema and constricting eschars add to the problems of direct respiratory insult. Gentle, thorough suctioning of the airway is frequently needed early to clear mucus and debris. In the patient with extensive secretions, endotracheal intubation or tracheostomy may be needed to keep the airway open. Constricting eschar of the chest may require escharotomy.

Burn patients have a tendency to vomit. If the mouth and face are swollen, the patient may not be able to handle the fluid. Aspiration can be a real danger.

Fluid therapy can contribute to the respiratory problems. Too much fluid can result in pulmonary edema, too little, in hypovolemia. If the patient becomes hypovolemic, tissue hypoxia can result in metabolic acidosis. Proper fluid balance, with maintenance of acid-base equilibrium, is essential.

The burn victim tends to have many factors contributing to hypoxia and to reduced respiratory tidal volume. Positive pressure breathing machines can be of great value when used judiciously. There can be a reduction in cardiac output before any significant alteration in circulating fluid volume. This, coupled with pulmonary insufficiency, can also result in tissue hypoxia.

The problems created by edema subside during the first week, as the patient reaches the diuretic phase. The threat of atelectasis secondary to bronchial occlusion resulting from necrotic slough and secretions continues. Thorough tracheal or bronchial toilet is essential to prevent this from happening. Bronchopneumonia may manifest itself any time after the first 3 to 5 days. The bacteria are introduced from the environment, and the weakened necrotic tissues provide fertile beds for the growth of organisms.

Respiratory acidosis may also be seen at this time. The patient may hypoventilate because of atelectasis, bronchopneumonia, or constricting eschar of the chest.

Many burn patients today are treated with topical mafenide (Sulfamylon) 10% cream. It contains a drug that acts as an inhibitor of carbonic anhydrase. If this enzyme is inhibited, sodium bicarbonate is excreted in excessive amounts through the kidney. The buffering effect of the sodium bicarbonate is then lost, and a metabolic acidosis can result. The patient compensates by hyperventilating. Usually this is only partially adequate. Additional sodium bicarbonate by mouth or by intravenous infusion is the usual means of restoring the acid-base balance to normal. Occasionally, the Sulfamylon treatment may have to be withheld for a day or two until the acid-base balance is restored.

Pulmonary emboli are an ever-present threat. Heat changes in the vasculature, sepsis, and the need for prolonged immobilization are all predisposing factors. Burn victims with a history of excessive smoking, asthma, pulmonary emphysema, or heart disease tend to do poorly. Young or elderly patients who cannot cooperate with coughing or rebreathing regimes also present many problems.

Proper management of respiratory problems in burns should include:
1. Oxygenation and humidification of the respiratory tract
2. Relief from upper airway obstruction caused by secretions and necrotic debris by careful tracheal toilet, endotracheal intubation, or tracheostomy
3. Use of respiratory support, such as positive pressure apparatus, if needed

4. Administration of adequate fluid therapy
5. Prevention of bacterial invasion by control of the environment and by proper sterilization of all equipment used for respiratory support
6. Judicious use of systemic and topical drugs for the control of bacteria

Current thinking is that respiratory problems rank with infection as the leading cause of death in burn victims.

## CHANGES IN THE HEART

The exact nature of the effect of burn injury on the heart is not fully understood. Cardiac output can decrease without significant alterations in circulating blood volume. Even in a patient with no prior history of heart condition, it is difficult to prevent fluid overload and resulting pulmonary edema. Digitalis preparations may be used to help support the heart function.

Bacterial invasion of the heart can occur as a result of sepsis. Patients treated with steroids are especially vulnerable. The hypertension seen in burned children has been correlated with the increase of excretion of urinary catecholamines.

## CHANGES IN THE LIVER

The necrosis or edema found in the liver after burn injury is felt to occur as the result of anoxia caused by a reduction in hepatic blood flow. This is related to general circulatory insufficiency. Liver physiology is altered. This can be related to the metabolic disturbances involving the utilization of energy, fats, carbohydrates, and protein. The details of liver function in burned patients await further research.

## CHANGES IN THE GASTROINTESTINAL TRACT

Gastric dilatation and paralytic ileus appearing early in the course of burn injury can be a direct result of the injury. They can also be neurogenic in origin, secondary to fear or pain, or can occur as a result of hypovolemia that results in splanchnic constriction. Sepsis is also a major cause of gastric dilatation and paralytic ileus. Gastric dilatation and ileus can occur at any time during the burn course.

The blood seen initially in the gastric secretions may result from gastritis. The bleeding may result from congestion of the capillaries of the gastric mucosa, which are delicate and rupture easily. This condition usually clears within a few days.

A gastrointestinal ulcer known as Curling's ulcer is also associated with burn injury. These ulcers can occur within a few days of injury or at a later time. Antacids and a bland diet help; occasionally, surgery is necessary.

## CHANGES IN THE KIDNEY

The kidneys can react to burn injury on a temporary or permanent basis. The level of the anatomic lesion can be either in the glomerulus or in the tubules. The temporary form is manifested by oliguria. With the loss of fluid circulating volume, there is renal vasoconstriction, which leads to an early decrease in glomerular filtration. The blood urea nitrogen and creatinine are elevated. The initial shock of injury may also stimulate the secretion of antidiuretic hormone from the posterior pituitary gland.

The glomerular filtration returns to normal if the patient receives adequate fluid resuscitation. If there is no history of prior kidney disorder, tubular damage is still possible, because of the circulation of breakdown products from the burn. This is particularly likely if inadequate fluid resuscitation has been used. By the third or fourth day of treatment there is readjustment of the fluid shifts and of the electrolyte balance. Sodium and chloride are reabsorbed, potassium is excreted, and water, creatinine, and urea are handled. The patient will undergo diuresis.

If there is a history of prior kidney disorder or if the patient does not receive adequate fluid therapy, permanent kidney damage may result. Permanent or persistent renal failure can be oliguric or nonoliguric. The latter type occurs more frequently.

Mannitol or urea can be used as an osmotic diuretic or renal flush. Sometimes an extra bolus of fluid is all that is necessary. Renal dialysis can also be used, but this has proved to be unnecessary in all but a few burns since the advent of vigorous fluid therapy.

The initial hematuria seen is the result of the destruction of some of the red cells at the time of burning. Intermittent hematuria can occur as partially destroyed red cells die and disintegrate.

Glycosuria may be found initially and clear spontaneously. Occasionally the syndrome of burn stress pseudodiabetes occurs. The high-carbohydrate, high-calorie diet prescribed for the burn patient may lead to pancreatic depletion. The symptoms are high urine output with high specific gravity. The patient is hyperglycemic. The urine shows glycosuria without acetonuria. There is marked dehydration and high hematocrit, and the nonprotein nitrogen and serum sodium and chloride are elevated. The condition eventually clears following administration of insulin and adequate water.

**REFERENCES**

Harrison, H. N.: Respiratory tract injury, pathophysiology, and responses to therapy among burned patients, Ann. N. Y. Acad. Sci. **150**(3):627-638, 1968.

Harrison, H. N., and Zikria, B. A.: Management of respiratory problems in burned patients, Mod. Treat. **4**(6):1263-1281, 1967.

Moncrief, J. A.: Burns of specific areas. In Artz, C. P., editor: A symposium on burns, J. Trauma **5**:278, 1965.

Munster, A. M., and Pruitt, B. A., Jr.: Recent advances in the management of burns, Med. J. Australia **1**:484, 1971. (Reprints available from Dr. A. M. Munster, Trauma Study Branch, U. S. Army Institute of Surgical Research, Brooke Army Medical Center, Ft. Sam Houston, Texas 78234.)

Phillips, A. W.: Pulmonary complications in burned patients, Bahama International Conference on Burns, Philadelphia, 1964, Dorrance & Co., pp. 7-21.

Phillips, A. W., and Cope, O.: Burn therapy, III. Beware the facial burn, Ann. Surg. **156**:759, 1962.

Phillips, A. W., Tanner, J. D., and Cope, O.: Burn therapy, IV. Respiratory tract damage (an account of the clinical, x-ray and post-mortem findings) and the meaning of restlessness, Ann. Surg. **158**:799, 1963.

Sevitt, S.: Burns, pathology and therapeutic applications, London, 1957, Butterworth & Co. (Publishers) Ltd.

# CHAPTER 4

# Local care of the burn wound

Many of the procedures and dressing techniques used for the local care of the burn wound are similar throughout the course of treatment. Modifications are sometimes necessary for the different types of wound and for different phases of its treatment.

Care of *partial-thickness wounds* is geared to minimizing infection. in order to prevent conversion to full-thickness injury. The healing epithelium must also be protected from mechanical trauma.

Slough and eschar must be removed as quickly as possible from *full-thickness wounds* without depleting the general condition of the patient, in preparation for permanent grafting procedures.

*Grafted areas* must be protected from mechanical trauma and slippage. Infection must be kept to a minimum, and the grafts must be kept free of blisters to ensure adherance to the recipient bed.

## TYPES OF CARE

There appear to be many different techniques for treating the burn wound. Close study reveals that the basic techniques are relatively few in number. The materials used for dressings, the medications used, the physical setting called for, and the timing of various procedures can vary greatly. The results, however, can be surprisingly the same, if these basic concepts are adhered to:

1. Keep the patient's general condition as stable as possible by meeting his physical and emotional needs.
2. Keep infection to a minimum.
3. Pursue an aggressive course of definitive care, with close attention to the details of a particular treatment.

The most commonly used techniques are described in the following pages.

## Exposure

The burn wound is exposed to the air in this treatment, since bacterial growth is theoretically minimized in the absence of moisture. Exposure treatment has been used intermittently for many years. Some physicians feel that this is the best way to handle organisms resistant to other forms of treatment.

The success of this form of treatment requires a great deal of careful nursing. The patient's environment must be carefully controlled as to temperature and humidity. The use of isolation technique is a must. The bed linen should be sterile. Single surface wounds can be handled easily, but circumferential wounds are more difficult, since they require frequent turning (every 2 hours) of the patient. Turning frames protected by non-adherent coverings are very useful in this situation.

In the partial-thickness wound, the dried exudate and injured tissue form a seal of varying depth, which protects the tissues underneath from further contamination. Pathogenic organisms can usually be grown from these crusts, but if the exposure treatment is successful they are kept to a minimum, and the body is able to cope with them. It is the degree of infection, not the presence of infection, that is important.

The crust should be inspected daily for cracks and any loose particles. Depending on its depth, the crust begins to separate in about a week, though some areas may take considerably longer. Any crust that can be removed without causing bleeding is lifted and cut away. In the clean partial-thickness wound a healed area is found under the crust. If infection occurs, full-thickness damage may result.

Full-thickness burns treated by the exposure method have a dry, leathery covering at first. Natural action of bacteria then causes the collagen fibers to disintegrate and the eschar begins to loosen. The loosened eschar is lifted and cut away each day. The exposed bed may be covered with a dressing at this time.

The physician may order the burned and unburned areas cleansed each day to remove excess exudate. Care must be taken to cleanse uninfected and cleaned areas so that they are not contaminated by infected areas.

Grafted areas treated by exposure can be inspected easily. They can be checked for slippage, and exudate occurring under the grafts can be easily removed. The patient must be carefully positioned and restrained to prevent dislodgment of the grafts. Grafts that slip can be replaced if they do not dry out too much. Donor sites heal very well if kept exposed and dry.

**Tubbing**

Tubbing the burn victim was in disfavor in the recent past. Originally, patients were immersed in various solutions for fairly long periods of time. The patients were more comfortable, but it was impossible to control infection.

As used for the most part today, patients are tubbed for much shorter periods, usually not more than 30 minutes. The solution used can be normal saline, plain water, or electrolytically balanced mixtures, or it can contain nonirritating cleansing agents. The patient's wounds can be thoroughly cleansed at various treatment stages, and the patient can be exercised. Dressings can be removed more easily. Tubbing facilitates the loosening of slough, and eschar, exudate, and topical medications. Debriding is done more easily at the time of the bath. The ideal tub is a tank with an agitator.

Care must be taken not to chill the patient. If there are dressings, the outer portion should be removed before placing the patient in the tub. The inner adherent dressings can be removed as they loosen while in the tub. The inner gauze over a fairly fresh grafted area may be left in place. The gauze over a donor area is also not disturbed unless it loosens. Loose gauze is trimmed away. If possible, the patient should be allowed to help himself. A wash cloth or a plastic-foam surgical hand scrub sponge held firmly in the hand of the patient can be very effective in cleansing wounds.

Properly managed tubbing can minimize the number of a patient's trips to the operating room for debriding and dressing changes. Tubbing just before surgery, if possible, can shorten the time in the operating room.

**Occlusive dry dressings**

Massive occlusive dry dressings are rarely used today. They are used in the pregraft and postgraft stage for limited areas. Eschar and slough separate more rapidly under dressings of this type. Control of infection can be a great problem if the dressings are left on more than a few days.

The dressing materials may vary, but they should have certain characteristics in common. The dressings are a complex. The innermost layer is usually a single layer of fine-mesh gauze fine enough to prevent in-growth of new epithelium but wide enough to allow exudate to escape from the wound surface. A dry, inner layer can be used over a sloughing area to help pick up necrotic material. A lightly lubricated gauze (water-soluble type lubricant) is best over newly grafted areas or healing wounds. Sometimes an antimicrobial agent is incorporated into this inner layer. The effectiveness of this is dependent on the duration of the time during which the agent is capable of bactericidal or bacteriostatic action.

The next layer of the dressing must be bulky and fluffy to absorb any wound exudate and to hold it away from the wound surface. The outer layer should be a stretch type bandage to hold the dressing firmly in place, but not so tight as to constrict.

Properly applied dressings help the patient feel more comfortable and can help minimize contractures.

### Wet dressings

Wet dressings can be applied effectively in a variety of ways and at all stages of wound care. Maceration must be avoided in the healing wound and over grafts.

Wet dressings can be very messy. The nurse may be tempted to use plastic coverings for protection. In a hypothermic patient, this might be safe. In a normal or hyperthermic patient, the warmth created by the plastic can increase bacterial activity, or cause maceration of healing tissue.

A dry covering should be used over the wet dressing to keep the patient more comfortable and to minimize water loss by evaporation. If the patient becomes hyperthermic, the dry cover is removed until the temperature is down. If the patient becomes hypothermic, more dry cover or heat lamps should be used.

The dressings must be kept wet. A variety of solutions can be used, ranging from normal saline to complex antimicrobial solutions. The solution used depends on the type of organism cultured from the wound.

An inner, single layer of gauze is helpful in debriding a wound or preparing a granulation bed for grafting. When used over fresh grafts, especially the lace type, this inner layer of gauze need not be removed at each dressing change.

The bulk of the dressing can be thick gauze pads (at least 24-ply) or multiple layers of stretch bandage. Ease of application and removal should be a guide in selecting the dressing material to be used. The dressing must be thick enough to hold sufficient fluid against the wound surface without too frequent wetting.

Complete dressing changes should vary with the amount of soiling. Keeping a soiled dressing wet is of little value.

### Topical antimicrobials

The concept of burn wound sepsis focuses attention on control of the number of organisms in the burn wound. Since the burn wound is avascular, proper use of topical medication is important in helping to control the number of organisms. The agents used should have these characteristics:

1. Be capable of diffusing through the burn wound
2. Be nontoxic locally and systemically
3. Be noninjurious to viable tissue
4. Be nonantigenic
5. Pathogenic organisms should not develop resistant strains during use
6. Be inexpensive, readily available, and easy to use

The agents are applied in solution using wet dressings, or they are dabbed on the wounds, or they are incorporated into creams or ointments. Unless they are water soluble, ointments have a tendency to hold in heat, to macerate tissue, and to retard the absorption of the antimicrobial agent. Creams are more commonly used. The medications can be applied directly to the wound surface manually, incorporated into single-layer dressings, or combined with occlusive dressings.

The single-layer gauze dressing used with the topical cream or ointment and secured by a single layer of stretch bandage or net type tube dressing is not considered an occlusive dressing. This type of dressing helps keep the topical medication against the wound so that the medication is not dislodged by the patient's movements. Some burn wounds have a very slippery surface. It is almost impossible, at times, to keep medication on the wound surface without this thin dressing. The areas dressed in this manner should rest on surfaces protected by fairly thick, fluffy, absorbent pads. Inexpensive paper pads are available. These pads help absorb the exudate away from the wound surface and help keep the patient tidier, whether sitting in a chair or lying in bed.

The choice of antimicrobial agent and the form or manner in which it is used are dependent on the characteristics of the burn wound and on the stage of care. In very deep burns, the agent must be capable of diffusing through the wound. The type of organisms cultured from the wound or bloodstream also influences the choice of agent to be used. Certain topical agents are more effective than others against a particular organism. A particular antimicrobial agent can be used in cream or ointment form, with or without dressings, when the wound is being cleaned up prior to grafting. A solution of the same agent may be used in wet dressings to prepare a granulation bed for grafting. Freshly grafted areas may be left free of all dressings and creams or dressed with creams or wet dressings.

Personnel must know the untoward symptoms that can occur with the use of a particular therapy. They must be aware of the objectives of care at

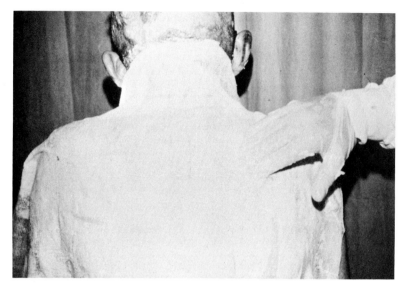

**Fig. 4-1.** Application of single-layer gauze dressing, impregnated with Sulfamylon acetate 10% cream. (Courtesy Dr. P. Stoddard.)

any stage of wound care. If the wound or the patient is not progressing properly, the "burn team" must be alerted so that treatments can be reviewed and perhaps modified.

The perfect antimicrobial topical medication has not yet been developed. There are many agents in wide use today; some are more popular than others. They all have their virtues and their limitations. It is most important to have a number of agents available and to be familiar with their characteristics. The most commonly used agents are discussed in the following paragraphs.

**Mafenide acetate (Sulfamylon) 10%.** Sulfamylon cream is especially effective for deep burns. It can diffuse through avascular burn tissue and so help control infection. The cream can be applied directly to the burn wound surface, using a sterile tongue blade, or by hand, using a sterile glove. The cream can then be left on the wound uncovered, or it can be covered by a single layer of fine-mesh gauze and secured by stretch gauze or tube net dressing. For small areas and hands, strips of fine-mesh gauze can be impregnated with the cream and laid on the wound surface. The cream must be applied so that the burn wound cannot be seen. The cream can also be incorporated into an occlusive dressing, if necessary.

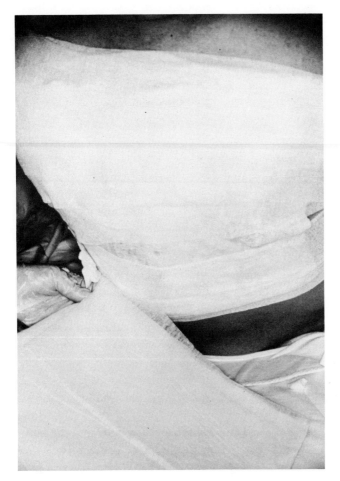

**Fig. 4-2.** Single-layer gauze dressing secured by stretch gauze. Burn underpad is placed in position to absorb any excess exudate when patient is lying on back. (Courtesy Dr. E. Parrish.)

The cream is usually applied twice a day and replaced as necessary, if it is rubbed off. The dry cream and exudate should be removed before reapplication. The cream has a tendency to cake, and tubbing is probably the best way to remove it. If tubbing is not possible, soaking the crusts with warm cleansing solution for at least half an hour will facilitate removal.

Because it is an effective inhibitor of a wide range of gram-positive and gram-negative organisms, Sulfamylon cream limits the quantity of bacteria

| | BURN - PERCENTAGE OF BODY SURFACE AREA | | | |
|---|---|---|---|---|
| | 1-39 | 40-59 | 60-79 | >80% |
| | ---------- MORTALITY - % ------------- | | | |
| PRE-TOPICAL ERA. N = 185 | 20-30 | 77 (WOUND SEPSIS - 45%) | 95 | 100% |
| SULFAMYLON (BROOKE, 1970) N = 257 | 3-5 | 43 (WOUND SEPSIS - 5.0%) | 81 | 100 |
| SILVER SULFADIAZINE (PARKLAND, 1970) N = 345 (ALSO USED SUBESCHAR + SYSTEMIC ANTIBIOTICS) | 3-5 | 25 (WOUND SEPSIS - 8.0%) | 45 | 93 |

**Fig. 4-3.** Burned patient topical therapy as of 1970. ( Courtesy Dr. H. Harrison. )

in the wound. The eschar therefore tends to take longer to slough, because eschar separation is dependent on the proteolytic action of bacteria. Any really effective antimicrobial agent will have this effect.

Sulfamylon has a tendency to cause a stinging sensation when first applied. The intensity of the reaction appears to vary according to the makeup of the individual. Full-thickness wounds should not be as painful as partial-thickness wounds. The pain associated with the full-thickness wound comes from sensation at the healing edges of the burn wound.

Sulfamylon is a carbonic anhydrase inhibitor and so may lead to impairment of the renal buffering mechanism. The resulting acidosis can be compensated for by the respiratory system. If there is impairment of the respiratory system, such as is caused by pneumonia, the patient may need additional sodium bicarbonate. Sulfamylon should not necessarily be stopped for that reason.

Some patients may show a rash, which must be reported to the physician. Antihistamines can be given. Patch tests should be made to determine that it is really the Sulfamylon that is causing the reaction.

**Gentamicin sulfate (Garamycin) 0.1% cream.** Garamycin is used in the same manner as Sulfamylon. The cream spreads much more readily and disappears rather quickly into the burn wound. There is no pain associated with its application.

Garamycin is effective against a wide range of gram-negative and gram-positive organisms. It is especially effective against the *Klebsiella* and *Enterobacter* groups. Because of the tendency of organisms to develop resistance to this drug, it behooves those using it to reserve it only for life- threatening situations.

Occasionally, nephrotoxicity or ototoxicity may be manifested when this drug is used.

**Silver sulfadiazine 1%.** Silver sulfadiazine 1% is a water-soluble ointment and is spread in a film 2 to 4 mm. thick. It can be applied directly to the burn wound by a sterile gloved hand and left exposed, or a single-layer mesh gauze dressing may be used to hold the ointment in place, or occlusive dressings may be used. The ointment is reapplied as it rubs off. If occlusive dressings are used, they may be left in place 48 hours. This ointment is frequently incorporated into dressings used to hold temporary and permanent grafts in place. Thorough cleansing of areas covered with this ointment is needed to remove the gray film that may form on the wound surface.

Silver sulfadiazine 1% ointment is particularly effective against *Pseudomonas* infections. The action of this drug is dependent on the chloride and other anions present in the wound exudate. Patients feel no pain from the effects of the ointment, but skin rashes may appear if the patient is sensitive to sulfonamides.

**Silver nitrate 0.5% solution.** Silver nitrate solution is incorporated into wet dressings that can be applied continuously on the burn wound and over grafts. The silver ion has an oligodynamic action on bacteria and is considered bactericidal in effect. This solution can only penetrate through 1 or 2 mm. of burn eschar; therefore, only surface bacteria on the wound can be controlled. Treatment must be started early, before deep colonization of the wound develops.

The wound and graft surfaces must be free of any oil or grease film in order for this solution to be effective. The dressings used must allow for complete diffusion of the solution to the wound surface. Dr. Carl Moyer advocated the use of six or eight layers of 4-ply all-gauze dressings, all thoroughly wet with the solution before application.

The dressings should be closely held to the wound by stretch bandages. The dressings must be kept thoroughly wet with the silver nitrate 0.5% solution at all times between dressing changes. The patient is covered with a dry blanket to minimize evaporation. The blanket should be changed if it becomes damp. Tubbing can be used in conjunction with these soaks. Debriding is done at the time of dressing changes.

Patients are usually quite comfortable with these dressings until the eschar is removed. Exposed areas of deep, partial-thickness burn are apt to be painful at the time of dressing change. No pain is felt in areas of full-thickness burn. The nurse should see that the patient is properly sedated.

Although true argyria symptoms are not a complication, potassium and sodium levels are depleted with the use of this method. Plentiful supplies of test tubes, needles, and syringes must be on hand to facilitate the taking of the many blood samples needed. During the acute stage of the major burn, there can be serious consequences if potassium and sodium levels are not checked frequently. While busy with other problems, the doctor may need a diplomatic reminder to make the check.

In children with burns of more than 10% of their body, these tests may be as often as every 4 hours. In adults with burns of more than 20% of body surface, the tests should be done every 6 to 8 hours. It is absolutely essential that patients receiving silver nitrate therapy be given supplemental calcium, potassium, and sodium chloride. These are given intravenously at first, and then orally as tolerated.

The use of silver nitrate soaks presents many problems for the nurse. Care of the dressings is time consuming. Everything that comes in contact with the solution becomes stained. Walls and equipment must be protected. Separate clothing and shoes should be kept for the burn room. Linen should be kept separate and laundered in special units. Gloves should be worn at all times to protect the patient and the hands of people caring for him. Warm soapy water helps remove some of the staining, but special stain removers are required. The success of Dr. Moyer's treatment in extensive and severly burned cases that are carefully monitored would seem to justify the hard work required.

A special warning is necessary here. If dressings become too dry, the solution becomes concentrated and may cause damage to underlying tissues.

Many other agents too numerous to mention are also used. More studies involving the ability of the various agents to truly control burn wound sepsis need to be done. Quantitative analysis of burn wound cultures taken before and during the course of antimicrobial treatment should be done. Directions given for the amount of topical agent to be used are too general, for the most part.

### Dab technique

The patient's wounds are exposed, and solutions of appropriate type, antiseptic or antimicrobial, are dabbed on the wounds, as ordered. As cracks appear in the eschar, the necrotic material is carefully trimmed away. Open areas are covered with fine mesh gauze. The patient must be turned frequently to prevent undue maceration of affected parts.

### Subeschar injection

The area under the burn eschar is cultured. Appropriate antimicrobial solutions are administered by means of hypodermoclysis into the subeschar area. This treatment is used in conjunction with the exposure method.

## ESCHAROTOMY

The eschar of the full-thickness wound can be leathery and inelastic. If the neck, chest, or abdomen is involved, the patient can have difficulty breathing properly. If eschar occurs circumferentially on an extremity, circulatory embarrassment can result. The tightening effects of the eschar can occur immediately, in a matter of hours, or sometimes after several days.

The incision only through the eschar to release the pressure is known as escharotomy. It can be a bedside procedure. The procedure should be painless, and there should be little bleeding. In some cases deeper incisions that extend into the fascia are necessary. This is called fasciotomy. There is apt to be bleeding and some pain with this procedure.

## ESCHAR REMOVAL

One of the most challenging problems in local care is the removal of the thick, leathery eschar of the full-thickness wound and the removal of the slough of the partial-thickness wound. The following procedures can be used to accomplish this.

### Debridement

Debridement is the removal of eschar at the interface of the living and dead tissue. This procedure can be done in the hydrotherapy tub, in the operating room, in the dressing room, or at the bedside of the patient. Only the dead tissue that can be cut free without causing too much bleeding is removed.

The blunt end of a scissors or forceps can be used as a probe and slid into openings in the eschar. Careful movements, working below the eschar, can loosen necrotic tissue. Vigorous tugging and jabbing of the eschar surface is not necessary. Debriding can be done with a minimum amount of sedation if properly managed. Extensive initial debriding, if done, is best handled in the operating room with the patient fully sedated.

Debriding can be done with a dermabrader, which uses sandpaper, or the eschar can be planed off with a dermatome. The dermabrader can be used to remove the necrotic tissue of the partial-thickness wound. When used with the full-thickness wound, it serves to clear away the loose, dead tissue that would impede the cutting edge of the dermatome.

When silver nitrate 0.5% solution is used, the physician may elect to plane the eschar down, if it is too thick. This solution penetrates only 1 or 2 mm. into the eschar. Better wound infection control is achieved this way.

Dry or wet dressings can also help to remove some of the necrotic material. Dry dressings are usually wet to facilitate their removal. If they are not wet too much, or if the wet dressings are allowed to dry a little just before removal, much necrotic matter can be lifted up.

### Excision

Excision is the removal of eschar by sharp dissection, usually to the fascial level. It is an operating room procedure, since there can be considerable loss of blood. Excision may be done initially or in stages.

**Initial excision.** Initial excision is done in the first week post burn. It is usually used on small areas (10% or less) of well-defined full-thickness injury. Permanent or temporary grafts are used for coverage. These grafts must be checked for hematoma formation. Any clots accumulating must be removed as soon as possible. Blood prevents the adherence of the graft to the underlying bed.

**Staged excision.** With staged excision, the eschar is removed in the first weeks after injury during multiple operative procedures. Permanent or temporary grafts are used to cover the wounds.

At the time excision is performed, the surgeon may decide that the wound does not look clean enough or that satisfactory hemostasis cannot be achieved. Autografts may be taken at the time of surgery in the operating room. They are then applied several days after surgery, when the wound is in a more satisfactory condition. This can be a bedside or a treatment room procedure.

### Tangential excision

Tangential excision is done to the point of capillary bleeding or pain. It may be done initially or in stages, before the wound becomes heavily colonized by bacteria. It can be an operating room procedure, or it may be done in a treatment room or at the patient's bedside. Temporary grafts, homografts, or heterografts can be used to cover the wounds.

Some necrotic material may be left on the wound surface. Dry or wet dressing changes and tubbing can be used for cleansing.

Because this form of excision may not be deep enough to remove all the epithelializing elements, some regeneration of epithelium may occur. When homografts or heterografts are used, they seem to stimulate this regrowth of epithelium. If autografts have been used, they will be rejected from areas that are reepithelializing.

This form of excision was used in the past, but its use has been renewed recently.

## PREPARATION AND CARE OF GRANULATION BEDS

As they develop and are exposed, granulation beds are best covered with a protective dressing. This can be a single layer of dry or lubricated fine-mesh gauze or a wet dressing complex. The fine-mesh gauze helps produce a flat, clean, granular surface before grafting. Small granulating areas remaining after grafting reepithelialize better if they are kept clean and flat, and scarring may be minimized.

Topical antimicrobial creams used on granulation beds are usually discontinued several days prior to grafting. Wet dressings are then used to prepare the bed. Temporary grafts are also used to prepare the granulation bed for final autografting.

### REFERENCES

Artz, C. P., and Moncrief, J. A.: The treatment of burns, Philadelphia, 1969, W. B. Saunders Co.

Cramer, L. M., McCormack, R. M., and Carroll, D. B.: Progressive partial excision and early grafting in lethal burns, Plast. Reconstr. Surg. **30**:595, 1962.

Fox, C. L., Jr.: Silver sulfadiazine—a new topical therapy for *Pseudomonas* in burns, Arch. Surg. **96**:184-188, 1969.

Harrison, H. N., Bales, H., and Jacoby, F.: The behavior of mafenide acetate as a basis for its clinical use, Arch. Surg. **103**:449-453, 1971.

Jackson, D. M.: Second thoughts on the burn wound, J. Trauma **9**:839-862, 1969.

Krizek, T. J.: Care of the burned patient; the management of trauma, Philadelphia, 1968, W. B. Saunders Co.

Monafo, W. W.: The treatment of burns; principles and practice, St. Louis, 1971, W. H. Green, Inc.

Moyer, C. A., and Butcher, H. R.: Burns, shock and plasma volume regulation, St. Louis, 1969, The C. V. Mosby Co.

Personal communications: H. Bales and W. Moore.

Stone, H. H., and others: Gentamicin sulfate in the treatment of *Pseudomonas* sepsis in burns, Surg. Gynec. Obstet. **120**:351-352, 1965.

# CHAPTER 5

# Initial burn care management

Hospital personnel tend to be overwhelmed when they are confronted with burn injuries. Perhaps this is because of the appearance of the victim. Actually, burn care is easy to institute because many of the initial problems can be anticipated.

Initial procedures can be standardized. A procedure book or outline for administering care to burn victims should be available to personnel in the out-patient clinic and in the hospital emergency room. Special forms, helpful in recording pertinent information, should also be available as needed.

## ESTIMATION OF BURN

The diagram shown in Fig. 5-1 utilizes the Lund and Browder method of estimating the area of body surface involvement. This method allows for the change with age in the percentage of the total body surface area represented by the head, thigh, and foreleg.

The "rule of nines" can also be used as a good estimation. With this system, the head and each arm are all figured at 9% each. The anterior and posterior trunk and each leg are figured at 18% each. The perineum is figured at 1%.

A very easy method of estimating a scattered burn is to compare the victim's hand with your own. Allowing for the difference in size, the hand accounts for approximately 1% of the body surface area.

## PRIORITIES OF CARE

For effective management, priorities of care must be followed. These are:
1. The burning process must be stopped. The victim may still be smoldering when presented for treatment.

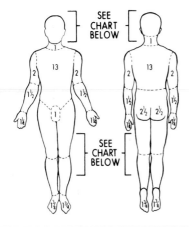

SEE
CHART
BELOW

SEE
CHART
BELOW

AGE :_____
SEX : _____
WEIGHT :_____
HEIGHT : _____

COLOR CODE
RED - Full
BLUE - Partial
GREEN - Available donor sites

| AREA | Inf. | 1-4 | 5-9 | 10-14 | 15 | Adult | Part. | Full | Total | Donor areas |
|---|---|---|---|---|---|---|---|---|---|---|
| HEAD | 19 | 17 | 13 | 11 | 9 | 7 | | | | |
| NECK | 2 | 2 | 2 | 2 | 2 | 2 | | | | |
| ANT. TRUNK | 13 | 13 | 13 | 13 | 13 | 13 | | | | |
| POST. TRUNK | 13 | 13 | 13 | 13 | 13 | 13 | | | | |
| R. BUTTOCK | 2½ | 2½ | 2½ | 2½ | 2½ | 2½ | | | | |
| L. BUTTOCK | 2½ | 2½ | 2½ | 2½ | 2½ | 2½ | | | | |
| GENITALIA | 1 | 1 | 1 | 1 | 1 | 1 | | | | |
| R.U. ARM | 4 | 4 | 4 | 4 | 4 | 4 | | | | |
| L.U. ARM | 4 | 4 | 4 | 4 | 4 | 4 | | | | |
| R.L. ARM | 3 | 3 | 3 | 3 | 3 | 3 | | | | |
| L.L. ARM | 3 | 3 | 3 | 3 | 3 | 3 | | | | |
| R. HAND | 2½ | 2½ | 2½ | 2½ | 2½ | 2½ | | | | |
| L. HAND | 2½ | 2½ | 2½ | 2½ | 2½ | 2½ | | | | |
| R. THIGH | 5½ | 6½ | 8 | 8½ | 9 | 9½ | | | | |
| L THIGH | 5½ | 6½ | 8 | 8½ | 9 | 9½ | | | | |
| R. LEG | 5 | 5 | 5½ | 6 | 6½ | 7 | | | | |
| L. LEG | 5 | 5 | 5½ | 6 | 6½ | 7 | | | | |
| R. FOOT | 3½ | 3½ | 3½ | 3½ | 3½ | 3½ | | | | |
| L. FOOT | 3½ | 3½ | 3½ | 3½ | 3½ | 3½ | | | | |
| | | | | | | TOTAL | | | | |

**Fig. 5-1.** Burn estimate diagram.

2. Respiratory needs must be determined. An adequate airway must be established.
3. Fluid needs must be met.
4. Care of the burn wound comes last.
5. If the patient is conscious, a feeling of security must be conveyed from the very first.

Adequate records must be kept, starting in the emergency room. Most of the equipment and supplies needed for the initial treatment of a burn victim are standard items in a hospital dispensary or emergency room. Even a very small facility should be able to handle a major burn victim until transfer to a burn unit or referral center is arranged. Proper organization of available equipment is essential.

The special dressings, topical medications, and sterile linen (if used) for burn care can be stocked in a special cabinet or on a shelf to be readily available if needed. A hospital facility confronted with a large number of burn victims has as its initial major concern the need for supplies to provide respiratory care. Provision for the administration and monitoring of fluids is next in importance. Burn wounds can be cleansed and dressed as personnel and materials are available. The patients should be kept as comfortable as possible with sedatives and kept dry and warm with any materials available.

The following outlines are suggested as guides for affording definitive initial treatment.

### BURN CARE EQUIPMENT INVENTORY

    I. Equipment and supplies for providing systemic care
        A. Appropriate attire
           1. Caps and masks
           2. Sterile gloves
           3. Operating room gowns (clean or sterile)
        B. Sterile drape sheets or towels
        C. Sterile water or sterile saline (tepid) for external use. Supply of ice and cooled fluids may be needed if patient is still smoldering.
        D. Equipment for respiratory care
           1. Tongue blade and flashlight
           2. Nebulizer for delivering moist air or oxygen
           3. Tracheostomy or endotracheal intubation setups
           4. Tracheal suctioning equipment

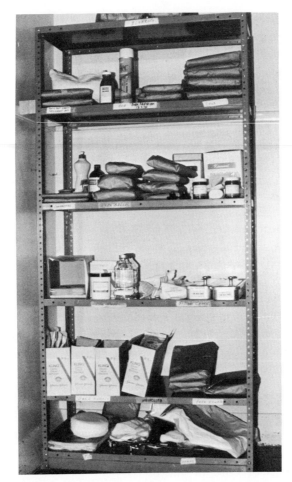

**Fig. 5-2.** Organization of equipment for admission of burn patient. (Courtesy G. Cher-nowitz.)

E. Equipment for fluid needs
1. Setup for establishing intravenous line (cutdown may be necessary)
2. Central venous line with manometer to be available if needed
3. Appropriate solutions for providing fluid needs
a. Colloid (Albuminsol)
b. Electrolyte (Ringer's lactate solution)
c. Free water (5% dextrose and water)

        4. Syringes, needles, and appropriate containers for collecting needed blood and urine samples
- F. Gastric tube connected to suction apparatus
- G. Urinary retention catheter connected to closed drainage system
- II. Equipment and supplies for providing wound care
  - A. Cleansing
    1. Hubbard tank or shower, if available, or moderately sized sterile basins for cleansing and rinsing solutions
    2. Tepid sterile water or sterile saline for external use
    3. Nonirritating cleansing agent
    4. Small all-gauze sponges
    5. Scissors and forceps (at least two sets)
  - B. Dressing materials
    1. Gauze rolls: dry or water-soluble cream type (Furacin)
    2. All-gauze dressings of various sizes
    3. Stretch type bandages
    4. Material for making splints
    5. Topical medication: Sulfamylon 10%; Garamycin 0.1% (gentamicin); silver nitrate solution 0.5%; silver sulfadiazine 1%

For determining the type of treatment facility needed, the following classification can be used.

## BURN CLASSIFICATION

*Minor burns*

Partial thickness or second degree
of less than 15%

Full thickness or third degree of
less than 2%

May be treated on out-patient basis

*Except in cases involving:* infants; elderly persons; face, hands, feet, or genitalia; possible respiratory involvement; prior cardiac, renal, or metabolic disorder; concomitant fracture or soft tissue injuries: *may need hospitalization*

*Moderate burns*

Partial thickness or second degree
of 15% to 30%

Full thickness or third degree
of less than 10%

Usually require hospital admission

*Except in cases involving:* infants; elderly persons; face, hands, feet, or genitalia; possible respiratory involvement; prior cardiac, renal, or metabolic disorder; concomitant fracture or soft tissue injuries: *may need to be considered in the major burn category*

Major burns

    Partial thickness or second degree of over 30%

    Full thickness or third degree of face, hands, feet, or genitalia; or more than 10% surface area involvement

    Burns complicated by:

        Prior cardiac, renal, or metabolic disorder

        Major soft tissue damage

        Fractures

        Electrical burns

        Chemical burns (especially alkali type)

        Infants or elderly persons

        Respiratory tract injury

All require hospital treatment and may need facilities of burn unit or burn referral center

## MANAGEMENT OF THE OUT-PATIENT BURN

1. All burned patients not requiring hospitalization need careful local care and followup to avoid the complication of infection.

2. Mask and sterile glove technique should be used for the initial burn wound dressing.

3. Wounds are gently cleansed with dilute, nonirritating soap solution. Special treatment is given for wounds caused by chemicals or tar.

    a. For chemicals, rinse thoroughly with appropriate neutralizing solution or copious amounts of water (see Chapter 12).

    b. For tar, apply ice or cold water. *Do not remove tar forcibly.*

4. Basic dressing should be fine-mesh, lightly lubricated gauze (water-soluble-type antiseptic or antimicrobial cream) covered with dry, all-gauze dressings, which provide suitable protection and absorptive capacity. Secure with lightly compressing stretch gauze bandage. Special treatment includes the following:

    a. Face and neck are exposed or antimicrobial cream applied.

    b. Hands are dressed and splinted in position of function.

5. Tetanus prophylaxis is mandatory unless a booster dose has been given within 1 year. If the patient has previously had at least two diph-

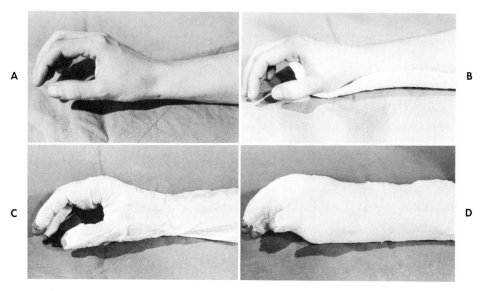

Fig. 5-3. **A,** Position of function. **B,** Proper placement of splint to preserve position of function. **C,** Application of single layer of gauze impregnated with Sulfamylon acetate 10% cream. Each finger is individually wrapped. **D,** Bulky, all-gauze dressing, with splint in place, secured by stretch gauze bandage. (Courtesy Dr. H. Bales and Mr. K. Elliott.)

theria, pertussis, and tetanus (DPT) injections, a booster of 0.5 ml. of DPT or 0.5 ml. of tetanus toxoid should be given. If the patient has not been previously immunized, immune human globulin (Hyper-tet) should be given.

6. The routine use of prophylactic systemic antibiotic therapy is not recommended. In selected cases, antibiotic therapy may be indicated.

7. An appropriate mild analgesic is prescribed.

8. Patient should be seen by physician within 48 hours.

9. On first visit 48 hours after receiving the burn, the dressing is checked for evidence of infection. Change is done at the discretion of the physician.

10. The first complete dressing change is advised within 5 to 7 days. All dressings, except the base layer of fine-mesh gauze next to the burn wound, are removed. If the fine-mesh gauze is dry and adherent, it is left in place. It will separate spontaneously as the reepithelialization of the superficial burn wound takes place. If soiled, it may be removed by soaking in a warm, non-irritating cleansing solution, and replaced with similar fine-mesh gauze lubricated with a water-soluble compound (not petrolatum). Culture and sensitivity specimen should be obtained if infection is present. Appropriate size all-gauze dressing and stretch type gauze roll ban-

dage are replaced. Subsequent dressings will be determined by the local wound. Change frequently (every day) if infected, less frequently if dry and clean.

### INITIAL MANAGEMENT OF THE HOSPITALIZED BURN PATIENT

1. Appropriate physicians should be notified (resident, attending).
2. Clean cap, gown, mask, and sterile glove technique should be used.
3. Use cold water and ice to stop the burning process, if necessary.
4. Airway must be secured immediately. Consider endotracheal tube or tracheostomy if respiratory distress is present. Oxygen therapy and humidity, and assisted ventilation are given as indicated.
5. Obtain brief history and record patient's weight.
6. Estimate percentage of burn surface area and record on burn diagram (see p. 39).
7. Intravenous route must be established (cut-down may be necessary) and appropriate solutions started. Unless there are other complicating factors, measurement of central venous pressure (CVP) is not always needed, and the CVP line need not be employed. Fluids should be given according to formula. The formula used must be modified according to parameters. Formulas are *only a guide* for projecting fluid needs.
   - A. After approximate needs are calculated the rate of fluid administration must be guided by frequent patient observation and laboratory tests, including:
     1. Clear sensorium
     2. Urine
        - a. Flow rate
           30 to 50 ml. per hour in adults
           20 to 30 ml. per hour in child above 2 years of age
           10 to 20 ml. per hour in child below 2 years of age
        - b. Specific gravity
        - c. Presence of hematuria
     3. Hematocrit
     4. Vital signs
   - B. Calculate fluid needs for the first 48 hours using a formula. The Brooke Army Formula utilizes 1.5 ml. electrolyte solution to 0.5 ml. colloid solution. The Evans Formula uses 1 ml. electrolyte solution to 1 ml. colloid solution. Both formulas include the use of free water according to age. The body weight (in kilograms) and the percent body surface area burned are used in making

calculations. Even if the body surface area involved exceeds 50%, usually 50% is used in making the calculation.

1. First 24 hours, Brooke Formula

Percent of burn surface area (BSA) × kg. body weight × 1.5 = ml. electrolyte solution (Ringer's lactate)

Percent burn surface area × kg. body weight × 0.5 = ml. colloid solution (Albuminsol)

2,000 ml. of 5% dextrose in water = daily free water requirement of an adult. The daily water requirement (milliliters of 5% dextrose in water to be administered) for children can be approximated as follows:

| | |
|---|---|
| Birth to 3 months | 700 ml. |
| 6 months | 1,000 ml. |
| 1 year | 1,200 ml. |
| 3 years | 1,300 ml. |
| 6 years | 1,400 ml. |
| 14 years and over | 2,000 ml. |

*One half of the total calculated fluid requirement for the first 24 hours after receiving a burn should be administered within 8 hours after injury (not dated from time of admission).*

2. Second 24 hours, Brooke Formula
   a. One half of day 1's calculated electrolyte solution
   b. One half of day 1's calculated colloid solution
   c. Daily water requirement as before
3. Subsequent days depend upon physiologic condition of patient, as indicated by observation, laboratory studies, amount of oral fluid taken, urine output, and specific gravity.

8. Administer adequate analgesic by intravenous (IV) route (Demerol, morphine sulfate). Calculate dosage according to age group and weight.

9. Gastric dilatation, vomiting, and ileus may complicate burn course. These can be managed with nasogastric suction and by restricting oral fluids.

10. Start a burn summary sheet (see Fig. 5-4). Record vital signs hourly.

11. Laboratory studies to be done as emergencies. These include:
    A. Complete urinalysis, including specific gravity, volume, culture, and sensitivity, and check for presence of blood
    B. Blood
       1. Type and cross-match
       2. Hematocrit
       3. Blood urea nitrogen

5D x 80 x 1.5

TIME OF BURN

| NAME | | | | | | | DAY POST BURN INJURY | | | | WEIGHT | | HEIGHT | | PERCENTAGE OF BURN | | | | | DATE | | |
|---|---|---|---|---|---|---|---|---|---|---|---|---|---|---|---|---|---|---|---|---|---|---|
| TIME | T | P | R | BP | CVP | HCT | ELECTROLYTE INSERTION SITE | HOURLY / TOTAL | COLLOID INSERTION SITE | HOURLY / TOTAL | D5W INSERTION SITE | HOURLY / TOTAL | URINE HOURLY / TOTAL | SPEC. GRAVITY | HEM | ph | PO or NG IN HOURLY / TOTAL | TYPE | NG OUT or EMESIS HOURLY / TOTAL | STOOL | HEM | REMARKS |
| 3 | | | | | | | lactated ringers rt. arm | | albuminsol rt. subclavian | | | | 100/100 | 1.030 | + | 6 | | | 0/0 | | | 10 mgm morphene sulfate IV push |
| 3 15 | 97 | 120 | 30 | 110/70 | 4 | 56 | // | 100/100 | // | 100/100 | | | 0/100 | | | | | | 0/0 | | | 0.5 Tet. Toxoid |
| 3 30 | | | | | | | // | 200/300 | // | 300/400 | rt. subclavian | | 0/100 | | | | | | 0/0 | | | |
| 4 | | 120 | 28 | 120/72 | 6 | | // | 200/500 | // | 0/400 | // | 100/100 | 50/150 | 1.029 | + | 7 | | | 120/120 | | | 5 mill. units penicillin IV push |
| 4 30 | | | | | | | // | 300/800 | // | 100/500 | // | 0/100 | 0/150 | | | | | | 0/120 | | | |
| 5 | 98 | 116 | 24 | 120/72 | 7 | | // | 200/1000 | // | 0/500 | // | 200/300 | 30/180 | 1.024 | 0 | 7 | | | 100/220 | | | |
| 6 | 98 | 110 | 24 | 120/70 | 7 | 50 | D-5 lactated ringers | 200/1200 | | 0/500 | | 100/400 | 40/220 | 1.024 | 0 | 7 | | | 0/220 | | | |
| | | | | | | | | | | | | | | | | | | | | | | |
| | | | | | | | | | | | | | | | | | | | | | | |
| | | | | | | | | | | | | | | | | | | | | | | |
| | | | | | | | | | | | | | | | | | | | | | | |
| | | | | | | | | | | | | | | | | | | | | | | |

**Fig. 5-4.** Burn summary sheet.

4. Prothrombin time
5. Electrolytes (sodium, potassium, carbon dioxide, chloride)
C. Nose, throat, stool, and wound culture.

12. Foley catheter should be placed in bladder and attached to closed drainage. Hourly measurement of urinary output is of vital importance. Check and record pH, specific gravity, presence of blood.

13. Check for constricting eschar on neck, chest, and abdomen (causing respiratory difficulties) and on extremities (causing lack of movement and sensation, poor capillary filling, and color changes).

14. Obtain chest x-ray.

15. Unless patient has a penicillin allergy, a penicillin preparation is indicated (as prophylaxis against β-hemolytic streptococci) during the first week of treatment. Thereafter, antibiotics are used as indicated by the clinical course. The choice of drug is based on specific culture and sensitivity studies, unless patient gives history of allergy.

16. Vitamins B and C are advised.

17. Give tetanus prophylaxis.

18. Photograph patient's wounds, if possible.

19. Care for the burn wound.

A. Shave hair from burn wound and from the area immediately surrounding it. Remove singed hair of the head by clipping. If the scalp, ears, or face are burned, the head should be shaved. Singed hairs falling into burn wounds can be very messy and cause itching.

B. Check eyes carefully. Ophthalmologic consultation may be necessary. Irrigate eyes with sterile saline and insert protective ointment. Singed eyelashes should be carefully trimmed.

C. Burned ears must be carefully cleansed with appropriate solution and debrided. Appropriate protective cream should be applied. Head must be positioned so that ears receive no pressure. Keep ear canals clean. Exudate and creams can cause troublesome ear pressure and infection, if allowed to accumulate.

D. Lips and mouth must be cleansed with appropriate solutions. An ointment is helpful in keeping lips lubricated.

E. Cleanse body wounds using tub or showering device if possible. Otherwise, use sterile basins filled with small gauze sponges and appropriate cleansing and rinsing solutions.

F. Remove separated epidermis. If blisters are firm, they can be left intact. If blisters are opened, they must be completely unroofed.

G. Treat clean wounds by wet or dry dressings, topical antimicrobial creams, or exposure.
1. Hands are dressed and splinted in position of function or as ordered.
2. Head and neck burns can be left exposed, dressed wet or dry, or covered with antimicrobial cream.
3. Perineal burns are usually left exposed but may need a dressing of antimicrobial cream or solution. Very frequent cleansing is necessary.

If the patient is extremely restless (such as in the case of an alcoholic patient) or if severe respiratory problems are anticipated, it is best to place the patient on a standard hospital bed initially. It is very difficult to control a restless patient on a turning frame. The patient can be transferred to a special turning frame, if necessary, as soon as his condition is stabilized.

If the patient is to be transferred to a burn unit or referral center, usually within a 48-hour period, he can be safely transported after initial definitive care has been given. It is most urgent that the receiving facility receive accurate information regarding the patient.

**REFERENCES**

Fox, C. L., Jr.: Burns, Curr. Pediat. Ther. 4:964-971, 1970.
Moncrief, J. A.: Burns methods of the U. S. Army Surgical Research Unit, Curr. Ther., pp. 739-748, 1966.
Personal communications: C. Davis, R.N., J. Mance, R.N., and S. Reynolds, R.N., and Drs. H. Bales, J. Morton, and R. McCormack.
Pruitt, B. A.: Management of burns in the multiple injury patient, Surg. Clin. N. Amer. 50(6):1283-1299, 1970.
Stone, N. H., and Boswick, J. A.: Profiles of burn management, Miami, 1969, Industrial Medicine Publishing Co.

# CHAPTER 6

# Nursing care of the burn patient

## GENERAL CONSIDERATIONS
### Time factor

The amount of time necessary to care for a burn patient depends on the burn phase (acute, management, or rehabilitative), the type and extent of injuries, the methods used for wound care, and the facilities and personnel available for giving care.

In the acute phase, nursing care may need to be continuous, on a one-to-one basis. If the facilities of an intensive care unit are not available, nurses trained in intensive care techniques may be needed. Very often two nurses, or a nurse and an assistant, are needed for some phases of acute nursing care.

On a very busy floor, private duty nurses with some experience in giving burn care can be used. If the nurse is not up to date in nursing techniques, more hindrance than help results.

In the management and rehabilitation phases, time for nursing care varies considerably. Is the patient bathed in the room or sent to hydrotherapy for tubbing? Are the dressings done by the physician, by a special dressing team, or by the nurse? How much can the patient do? Because of the many variables, it is difficult to make set statements regarding nursing time needed. Each case must be evaluated individually.

It has been suggested that approximately 7 to 12 hours of nursing time per patient per day is the average requirement.

### Medications

While medications are ordered by the physician, certain types are needed by the burn patient almost routinely. The nurse should review the initial medication orders; a diplomatic reminder to the physician may save much time and discomfort for the patient. These medications include:

1. Vitamin preparations, especially B and C
2. Analgesics or sedatives
3. Bowel softeners or laxatives
4. Antipyretics
5. Antacids
6. Antipruritics

Systemic prophylactic antibiotic preparations are used initially by many physicians during the acute phase of burn care; usually this is a penicillin preparation. During the management phase of care, antibiotics are given according to the results of cultures taken.

Medications, especially antibiotics, must be reviewed carefully to be sure that they are given only for the correct length of time. If habit-forming drugs are given for the control of pain, the possibility of the patient becoming addicted must be considered.

### Scheduling meals and sleep

Treatments should not interfere with the patient's meal periods, if possible. Burn patients have a tendency to complain that they are not allowed enough time for rest and sleep. This is often true. At times it may be necessary to keep a record of the amount of sleep the patient actually gets in order to plan schedules.

### Environment

In a hospital that does not have a burn unit, the burn patient is best managed on a surgical floor, in a private room if possible. More than one patient can be in the same room if they are in the same stage of their care. If protected by occlusive dressings or antimicrobial topical therapy, patients can be kept on open wards. In the acute phase, the patient may need to be in an intensive-care unit.

The physical environment in which the burn patient is kept can vary greatly. Patients kept in elaborate isolation units may not ultimately fare any better than those kept in open wards. Reverse isolation procedures can be used for patients kept in private rooms and intensive care units. If isolators are used, they must allow for easy access to the patient.

In evaluating the type of enviroment needed, one must keep in mind that even with modern antimicrobial therapy burn wounds can be a source of contamination. The presence of infection is to be expected; it is the degree

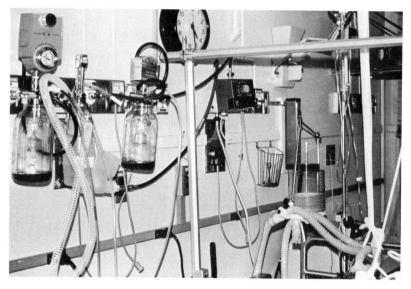

**Fig. 6-1.** Facilities for oxygen and gastric and tracheal suctioning. (Courtesy Dr. P. Stoddard.)

of infection that is important. Outside contaminants must be kept to a minimum.

The ideal setting for the burn patient is one in which the temperature and humidity can be controlled and the air filtered. Heat lamps should be available. Facilities for giving oxygen and for gastric and tracheal suctioning should also be available.

## Bed

The type of bed on which the burn patient is put is most important. A turning frame is best for a major burn. Nursing care is facilitated because wounds are more readily treated and the patient can be maintained in better position.

There are some very specialized bed units available. Some of these suspend the patient for a period of time on jets of air; others float the patient over water or plastic pellet material. For the most part, these special beds are in the experimental stage and tend to be expensive and cumbersome.

Net frames, which allow air to reach the patient's wounds, or frames that allow for bowel care can be used over a regular mattress. If regular mattresses are used, they must be well protected with waterproof covers.

Foamed paddings that can be easily laundered or discarded can also be used under the patient. Alternating pressure mattresses used over the regular mattress can minimize the development of pressure areas.

## Bed linen

Is sterile bed linen necessary? This is a subject of much debate. If linen can be secured with minimum handling within an institution, sterilization might not be necessary. If linen is handled many times, it can be a source of contaminants and should be sterilized.

If the exposure treatment is used, sterile linen is required. It may be used until the wounds are closed or grafting is completed. Most institutions using topical antimicrobial therapy do not feel that sterile bed linen is necessary. Some use sterile linen or sterile burn underpads only on the surface with which the open wound comes in contact.

Nonadherent absorbent pads, referred to as burn underpads, are very important items in caring for the burn patient. They are placed over the surface on which the burn wound rests. They help keep topical medications in place against the wound, yet they can absorb excess moisture and hold it away from the burn wound surface. They can also be protective in that when the patient is turned, the skin surface will not adhere to the bed sheeting. If the pads do become adherent they can be moistened for easy removal.

Thick gauze pads backed with a paper liner are good but fairly expensive. A thick paper pad or disposable diaper can be equally effective and cost much less. These pads must be changed frequently.

## Protective clothing for personnel

There is considerable variety in the clothing worn by personnel involved in giving burn care in the major burn units today. Common sense, combined with a knowledge of aseptic principles and the nature of the burn wound course, should help determine what is best. Because the burn wound is invariably infected, the staff as well as the patient must be protected.

## Head coverings

Protective head coverings are important for personnel. Hair brushing against the patient can be contaminated or can serve as a contaminating agent.

**Masks**

β-Hemolytic *Streptococcus,* which is commonly found in the nasopharyngeal tract, can be a real threat to the severely burned patient. The use of masks can minimize this. If masks are not used routinely, they should be worn when doing dressing changes and in the acute phase of care, when almost constant close contact with the patient is needed.

While the time period in which masks are effective varies considerably and is the subject of much debate, one point is clear: Discard mask as soon as possible after completion of patient contact. Do not suspend from neck and reuse.

**Clothing**

Special clothing is almost universally used in burn units. Some personnel shower before changing into the clothing worn on the unit. In a general hospital setting, this may not be feasible.

Protective clothing of some type, such as a precaution gown, is a must from the esthetic viewpoint, even if it is not used solely for the protection of the patient. One can argue for the patient's protection, but burn wounds can be very messy and the clothing of personnel could be very readily soiled.

If possible, special clothing that personnel can change into should be provided for those in constant attendance. Burn work can be strenuous. If the temperature of the room is kept so that the patient is comfortable (above 75° F.) people working in the room are apt to become uncomfortable if they wear a protective gown over a regular uniform.

**Gloves**

Clean gloves may be worn when giving direct patient care. Sterile gloves are used when doing dressings. Thorough hand washing is an absolute must before and after giving patient care if gloves are not used.

**Shoe covering**

The value of protective shoe covering is questioned. Many burn units require that personnel have shoes that are worn in the burn unit area only; others provide protective cloth, paper, or plastic shoe coverings. In a general hospital, shoe coverings can be provided if deemed necessary. Visitors as well as personnel must adhere to the protective clothing regulations adopted.

**Organization of equipment**

The equipment needed for individual care can be quite extensive. If possible, a special cart should be provided and kept near the patient's room. Suggested items for this cart are:

1. Masks, protective gowns, caps, and shoe covers, if used
2. Linen
3. Dressing materials
4. Solutions

## PLANNING FOR INDIVIDUALIZED NURSING CARE

Nursing care of the burn patient is facilitated if a careful evaluation of the patient is made. An individualized nursing care plan, based on the patient's needs and the physician's orders, is essential. The physician must be very specific when writing orders. Nursing care plans must be up to date and accurate records kept, so that each shift can have complete reports for the oncoming shift. Nursing care plans should cover the following important points.

**Vital statistics.** In the acute phase of burn care, hourly checks of vital statistics are necessary. This can be modified to 2- or 4-hour periods as the patient improves. During the management phase, because burn patients tend to be labile, checks should be done at least four times a day, or whenever a change in the patient is observed.

**Weights.** Daily weights are important during the first few weeks of care. Thereafter, patients should be weighed at least once a week.

**Output and input.** If a urinary catheter is in place, care must be taken to see that it is in proper position and that the drainage tubing is not twisted, thus impeding the urine flow. Irrigation may be necessary to flush out blood clots.

The urine must be measured for volume, pH, and specific gravity; checked for the presence of blood; and the results recorded. The indwelling urinary catheter can be removed as soon as the fluid replacement therapy is effective. If allowed to remain in place, it should be changed at least once a week. If catheter irrigations are ordered, they should be done only after the tests just mentioned are done. Careful cleansing of the urinary meatus is also required.

The insertion sites of intravenous equipment must be carefully checked for signs of infection and should be redressed at least once a day. During the entire course of treatment the nurse must continue to keep very accurate records of all fluid intake.

All intravenous and oral feedings must be carefully recorded. During the acute phase, special forms should be used (see burn summary sheet, p. 47).

When gastric suctioning is used, it is often difficult to keep the tube anchored, especially if the face is burned. Paper tape is a good anchoring material. The stomach contents should be carefully measured and tested for blood and the results recorded.

When the gastric tube is used for feeding purposes, the gastric residue should be checked before each feeding. The aspirate should be checked from time to time for the presence of gross blood. Gastric tubes left in place for long periods of time can cause erosion of the gastric wall. The gastric tube should be flushed carefully after each feeding.

**Respiratory care.** If there is respiratory involvement, the head of the bed should be kept elevated, and great care must be taken when turning the patient for the first time. Provision must be made for resuscitation, if needed. An intubation or tracheostomy set should be on hand.

If a tracheostomy is in place, a nebulizer is the best way to keep the mucous membranes moist. Separate sterile disposable catheters should be used for nasal or tracheal suctioning. The tracheal catheters are used only once. Vigorous tracheal suctioning must be avoided since the tracheal epithelium may be damaged. Mucolytic agents or sterile normal saline inserted into the trachea just before suctioning can help in removing thick secretions. Even if the patient sounds dry, suctioning may be needed.

Since the secretions may be very profuse and thick, the inner cannula needs frequent removal and cleaning. If a cuffed tube is used, the cuff must be deflated at regular intervals to prevent necrosis of the tracheal cartilage.

**Wound care.** See Chapter 4.

**Care of the mouth, eyes, and ears.** Good oral hygiene is important. It is frequently difficult for the patient to open his mouth. An irrigating syringe with a soft rubber tip can be used to flush the mouth; swabs or a soft small toothbrush may also be used. A cream or ointment can be used to soften the lips and keep them clean.

The eyes must be kept clear of exudate by careful cleansing and protected by ointment, as ordered. They should be kept as free of crusts as possible. If the ear is involved, it must be protected from further pressure damage by proper positioning. The ear canal should be checked frequently for exudate accumulation and cleansed as necessary.

**Care of unburned areas and healed burn wounds.** The unburned areas must be carefully cleansed. Exudate from the burn wounds may cause irritation if allowed to accumulate. If the patient is tubbed frequently, the skin has a tendency to become very dry. Lubricating lotions or creams are necessary to keep the unburned areas or healed wounds soft.

Pressure sores can be very difficult to avoid because of the necessity of prolonged immobilization and the weight losses suffered by the patient. The use of turning frames or foamed mattresses or padding can prevent and minimize some of these problems.

**Positioning.** Proper positioning of the burn patient is most important. Healing can be promoted and contractures minimized. Turning frames and foamed mattresses or paddings are all helpful.

Skeletal traction or special slings are also used for proper positioning and for facilitating wound care. Skin surfaces should not touch each other. When possible, involved areas should be positioned so that they do not touch the bed surface. Nonadherent pads or sheets, which can absorb exudate away from the wound surface, should be used if involved areas touch a surface.

It is essential that proper positioning be started at once and maintained until recovery. The neck should be kept hyperextended if the face, neck, or chest areas are burned. A short mattress placed over the regular mattress can be used. The patient's head rests on the lower mattress. A special mattress with an opening at the top cut in the shape of a half-moon can also be very useful in keeping the proper position.

If skeletal traction or slings are not used, extension for the knees should be as complete as possible, regardless of burn location. A foot board should be used to maintain the ankles in 90-degree flexion. The trunk and hips are maintained in anatomic position. The shoulders are also kept in anatomic position except when the axilla is burned. If this is the case, the arm should be immobilized in a 90-degree angle. One hundred forty degrees of flexion is suggested for elbow joints unless there is a burn in the antecubital fossa. If there is, complete extension is recommended because of the danger of contracture.

The positioning of the hands is of the utmost importance. There is a great deal of variance in the techniques used to preserve the shape and function of the burn-injured hand. Some physicians think that it is most important to keep the hand mobile. They use no dressings, just apply antimicrobial cream to the wound surface. Others enclose the hand in a medicated mitt type dressing that allows for frequent active and passive exercising. Still others think that an occlusive type dressing combined with a splint is necessary. The positioning of the wrist and hand also can vary a great deal.

In the postgraft stage, a dynamic type splint may be used. The nurse, the physial therapist, and/or the occupational therapist must ascertain exactly the position that the physician wants maintained. Dressings and splints must be applied in such a manner that the position ordered is maintained.

On p. 44 the occlusive hand dressing used to maintain the position of function is described and illustrated. This basic wound dressing is frequently used. The type of splint, the thickness of the dressing, and the positioning of the hand and wrist would be varied according to the physician's direct order.

Whenever possible, the burn patient is encouraged to be out of bed. For the patient covered with topical agents, single-layer gauze dressings secured with stretch bandages will help keep the topical medications in place. Wounds treated by exposure should be protected by nonadherent coverings, such as the paper burn underpad, so that sheets or clothing do not become adherent. Legs that have been burned must have the additional support of elastic type dressings.

Burn patients, especially those immobilized in bed for a long time, have a tendency to feel faint. The wound areas look purplish and tend to bleed easily, thus helping upset the patient. The patient must be reassured that the discolorations will subside and that some bleeding is expected, both when wounds are fresh and when they are healing.

Legs should be elevated on a foot stool if the patient sits in a chair for any period of time.

**Exercises.** Exercising may be done in the room or in the physiotherapy department. If trained therapists are not available, nursing personnel can help maintain joint mobility, under the physician's direction. The consensus today is that active motion exercises are more beneficial than passive ones. Trapeze devices on an overhead frame are very useful if the patient has the use of hands and arms and is allowed to move.

If special splinting devices are used, they must be kept clean. The skin areas on which the splint rests must be checked frequently for signs of infection, irritation, or erosion.

**Bowel care.** Stools must be observed for frequency and consistency. They should also be checked for the presence of blood. Fecal impaction must be avoided. With all the other problems in burn care, it is all too easy to overlook the bowel. Bowel softeners are helpful.

Burn patients have a tendency to develop diarrhea. Highly concentrated

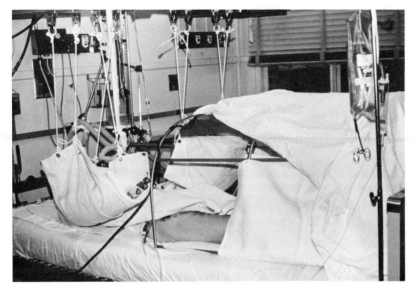

**Fig. 6-2.** Use of heated cradle and overhead frame to support arm slings. (Courtesy Dr. P. Stoddard.)

liquid feedings may be one of the causes. Oral antibiotics and some antacid preparations can also cause diarrhea.

If grafting of the buttock or upper thigh area is involved, at least 5 days before surgery a low-residue diet should be instituted to help minimize fecal contamination. A thorough cleansing enema before surgery is essential.

**Control of pain.** Pain-relieving drugs and tranquilizers should be used generously but judiciously, so that the patient is not in an aura of pain. Narcotics should be used only sparingly because of the long-term nature of the healing process. Care must be taken not to oversedate the patient to the point of interfering with mobility and oral intake.

**Nutritional support.** The need for proper nutrition is extremely important; Chapter 8 is devoted to a discussion of it.

**Use of special devices.** Heated bed cradles are helpful in keeping the patient warm and in keeping bed sheets off wound areas. Donor sites may heal faster when exposed to a heat lamp. If fresh grafts are exposed, they must be shielded so that they do not dry out too rapidly. If heated bed cradles are not available, heat lamps can be used to keep the patient more comfortable. They must be carefully positioned so that a burning hazard is not created.

Foot boards must be well padded if used for positioning. They must allow for foot support but not exert undue force on the soles of the feet.

Mirrors should be used, when available, to help the patient who must be kept flat to see the surrounding area. Bedside tables that enable the patient to do things independently should also be used when possible.

If a patient has trouble with feeding because of arm involvement, plates with protective rims to keep food from sliding off the plate and special cutlery will enable the patient to eat independently.

Toothbrushes, combs, and other implements needed by the patient can be adapted for use.

**Cultures.** Because infection is one of the leading causes of death from burn injury, frequent cultures are done. Initially the wounds, nose, tracheal secretions, stool, and urine are cultured. The blood is cultured only if the patient becomes hyper- or hypothermic. At the time the blood is cultured, cultures should also be repeated on the aforementioned secretions. Wound cultures are done at the discretion of the physician.

If an area becomes suspect, it should be reported to the physician. If *Pseudomonas* toxemia is suspected, urine can be tested for verdoglobinuria. The urine will show an olive fluorescence when examined under ultraviolet light in a darkened room if *Pseudomonas* is present.

Close clinical observation of the patient's physical status is as important as the taking of cultures. The patient must be observed closely for temperature changes (high or low), disorientation, gastric or abdominal distention, malaise or restlessness, vomiting, anorexia, and changes in wound appearance, such as disintegration of grafts or darkening of wounds.

**Psychologic support.** A great deal of time and effort can be saved if the following basic fact is kept in mind: prior to the closure of the burn wound by primary healing or by the use of grafts (temporary or permanent), the true personality of the burn patient does not manifest itself. Prior to the closure of the burn wound, therefore, supportive help is needed and should be started at the time of admission. Definitive psychologic therapy, if needed, is most effective when wound healing is nearly complete.

Severely burned patients are often not aware of the extent of their injuries. Some of them may even be euphoric. The less severely burned patient (partial-thickness wounds) may be in a great deal of pain. Pain and fear may cause the initial behavior problem.

During the acute and management phases of care, physiologic derangements caused by lack of oxygen, too little or too much fluid therapy, or electrolyte imbalances can contribute to the restlessness seen.

Many burn victims are alcoholic or addicted to drugs. Symptoms of withdrawal may contribute to the behavior seen. Epilepsy or a psychologic disturbance may have been present before the injury.

During the management phase, the patient may become very emotional or depressed. Painful treatments, fear of disfigurement, worry about financial needs, and guilt are just a few of the factors that can contribute to the patient's general upset. The intensity of the patient's reactions depends to a great extent on previous emotional makeup, adjustment to life, and extent of injury.

The patient must be guided to focus away from constant contemplation of self. Radio and television can be invaluable. The patient needs a great deal of verbal reassurance and explanation. Personnel in contact with the patient must always maintain a friendly but firm attitude. All the members of the burn team are needed to sustain the patient through the sometimes very long ordeal resulting from the effects of burn trauma. Comprehensive planning for discharge and followup are often necessary to help the patient in adjustment to normal living.

Personnel caring for burn patients, as well as the families involved, may need psychologic support. Personnel well grounded in the theory and practice of burn care usually do well. Physical good health, strength, and emotional stability are essential, because burn work can be very taxing physically and mentally.

Personnel assigned to burn care should be rotated off the service at least every 6 weeks, if possible, or reassigned to burn patients requiring different levels of care. In a general hospital, staff nurses should be assigned to an individual patient for at least a week, if possible. Too many changes will often upset the patient.

When private duty nurses are employed, they must sometimes be reminded to take time off. There is a tendency to become compulsive when caring for severely burned individuals.

Families may need the guidance of social workers to help them adjust. They may need monetary help as well as moral support. Families must also be enouraged to help in providing moral support for the patient. If they are made aware of the many problems involved, they are usually most cooperative. Members of the clergy and friends can be a source of great help in patient and family adjustments.

**REFERENCES**

Archambeault, C., and Feller, I.: Burn infection, J.A.H.A. **44**:118-120, 1970.
Artz, C. P., and Moncrief, J. A.: The treatment of burns, Philadelphia, 1969, W. B. Saunders Co.

Brantl, V. M., Brown, B. J., and Mooreland, M.: The care of patients with burns, comprehensive nursing care, Nurs. Outlook 6(7):383-385, 1958.

Decker, R., and Memec, B. M.: The care of patients with burns, convalescent and rehabilitation care, Nurs. Outlook 6(7):386-387, 1958.

Evans, E. B., and others: Prevention and correction of deformity after severe burn, Surg. Clin. N. Amer. 50(6):1361-1375, 1970.

Fay, N. C., and Dames, L. C.: Care of severely burned patients. In Bergersen, B., and others: Current concepts in clinical nursing, St. Louis, 1967, The C. V. Mosby Co.

Hoopes, J. E.: Recovery from burns, the management of trauma, Philadelphia, 1968, W. B. Saunders Co.

Jacoby, F.: A basic guide to burn nursing, Prize winning thesis, Rochester, N. Y., 1969, Rochester Academy of Medicine.

Minckley, B. B.: Expert nursing care for burned patients, Amer. J. Nurs. 70(9):1888-1893, 1970.

Stone, N. H., and Boswick, J. A.: Profiles of burn management, Miami, 1969, Industrial Medicine Publishing Co.

Watts, J.: Treatment of circumferential trunk burns by air on the inverted hovercraft principle of levitation, Bahama International Conference on Burns, Philadelphia, 1963, Dorrance & Co.

# CHAPTER 7

# Wound closure

## HEALING
### Partial-thickness wounds

Histologic studies show that wound healing occurs in several stages, provided that massive infection, mechanical trauma, or obliteration of the blood supply to the part does not intervene. During the first stage of the healing process, the fluid exudate brings to the wound leukocytes, histiocytes, and macrophages. These cells and the proteolytic enzymes also present aid in breaking down any dead tissue present.

By the second or third day fibroblasts and capillaries appear in the wound. By the fourth day, the fibroblasts have for the most part replaced the inflammatory cells. By about the fifth or sixth day, fibroplasia becomes quite extensive; this may result in scarring. The scar tissue later contracts, resulting in a decrease in capillaries and interstitial fluid.

Epithelialization proceeds quite rapidly if it is not impeded by necrotic tissue. This new epithelium develops from the vestiges of the epidermal appendages that may remain or from the edges of the wound. Reconstitution of the upper epidermis continues after resurfacing of the epithelium is completed.

New reticulin and collagen fibers are laid down in the demis. At first, this new dermis may not have a papillary layer. Elastic tissue may not reappear for some months. The viable epidermal appendages grow upward with the thickening dermis, but these areas may be deficient in those structures previously mentioned. Nerve endings are the last to regenerate. Sometimes improvement is noted over several months and even years.

The ability of the skin to resurface itself with epithelium is directly dependent on the depth of burn damage.

### Full-thickness wounds

Full-thickness wounds cannot reepithelialize; granulation tissue forms instead. This process proceeds in the following manner. When a burn wound creates a crater-like defect, the defect will gradually fill in with new connective tissue from its base and sides. Fibroblasts and capillaries grow into the moist exudate that fills the defect. A new, thin layer of exudate forms continuously as the granulation tissue bed is built up. Capillary arches forming in the growth surface cause the granular appearance of the tissue.

Small elevations of fibroblastic tissue and exudate form at each point where there is a prominent capillary arch. The healthy defect produces a red, richly vascularized, moist surface with a slightly granular appearance. This is known as granulation tissue. Capillaries within the granulation tissue tend to be very fragile and bleed at the slightest trauma. Infection will hinder development of granulation tissue. If not covered by epithelium, granulation tissue becomes overgrown or exuberant.

Preparation of large granulation beds for autografting is a very important facet of burn care. Resurfacing of small granulation areas from the edges of the wound can be greatly facilitated with proper wound handling.

In spite of excellent care, certain individuals, especially Negroes, have a tendency to develop large elevated masses of connective tissue. Resurfacing with epithelium does not appear to minimize the growth, which is referred to as keloid growth. Ordinary hypertrophic burn scars tend to soften and regress with time and to become lighter in color. Keloids continue to grow unless treated definitively by surgery or hormone therapy.

## GRAFTING

### Purpose

When all the epithelial elements are lost, as in full-thickness burn injuries, skin grafts are necessary to restore the body to its normal equilibrium and functions. Grafting in the management stage of burn care is done as soon as possible to minimize infection, fluid losses, and loss of function. Grafting in the rehabilitative stage is done to restore cosmetic appearance and to achieve maximum function and is best delayed for good results.

### Graft sources

*Autografts* are grafts obtained from the patient's own body. *Isografts* are histiocompatible tissues obtained at the present time principally from the victim's identical twin, if he is fortunate enough to have one. Isografts and autografts afford permanent coverage.

*Homografts* (or allografts) are obtained from the bodies of living or dead persons having suitable tissue (free from disease). *Heterografts* (or xenografts) are skin coverings from animal sources or of man-made materials. The principal animal sources are bovine, canine, or porcine tissue. Synthetic films of Teflon, nylon-velour, and polyurethane foam have been used. Homografts and heterografts afford only temporary coverage.

### Graft function

**Permanent.** The autograft and isograft must not only cover the burn wound to restore the body to normal equilibrium and function but must also restore the cosmetic appearance of the patient, if possible. The ultimate rehabilitation of the patient to normal living depends on this.

**Temporary.** Temporary grafts are used until a patient's own skin is available. Grafts utilizing synthetic materials have only a limited use, because infection can develop under them very rapidly. Their principal function is to prevent water evaporative loss.

Other temporary grafts can afford many benefits to the patient. They can reduce loss of water electrolyte and water protein at the burn surface. The reduction of water evaporative loss also lowers the caloric loss. The patient has less pain when the open wounds are covered and can move more easily. Being able to move improves the patient's morale. The patient has a better appetite, which helps build up his strength.

Temporary grafts are also thought to diminish infection in the burned area. Granulating areas can be kept in good condition until permanent grafts are available. If the physician is in doubt as to whether a recipient bed is ready for permanent coverage, the temporary graft can be used as a means of determining take.

Burns of questionable depth or deep dermal burns may be covered with temporary grafts after eschar or burn slough is debrided. The grafts seem to stimulate the epithelial elements, and the wounds heal better. In cases where complications such as pneumonia or gastric hemorrhage occur, permanent coverage can be delayed until the patient is in condition for surgery. Temporary grafts may then be left on until rejected by the body (a matter of weeks).

When used to test the receptivity of the granulation bed to autograft or to control infection, temporary grafts are removed after only a few days or daily so that they do not become too adherent. They can then be replaced readily, as necessary.

### Graft types

There are two basic types of skin grafts: the split-thickness skin graft and the full-thickness skin graft. These grafts are possible because skin can remain alive for a short period of time without blood supply. Apparently there is an osmotic interchange with the intercellular fluid of the recipient bed, which nourishes the graft until capillary invasion from the recipient bed establishes the blood supply.

**Split-thickness grafts.** The split-thickness graft can vary in thickness from 0.008 to 0.020 inch. The thinner split-thickness graft (sometimes referred to as the Ollier-Thiersch graft) has a better take than the thicker graft. The thickness of the graft depends on the amount of dermis taken. The thicker grafts (sometimes called intermediate or three-quarter thickness grafts) give much better cosmetic appearance. In the management phase of burn care the split-thickness graft is the most commonly used type and is applied as follows.

*Pinch graft.* A small piece of skin is elevated with forceps, cut from the donor site, and placed on the recipient bed. This kind of graft is becoming obsolete.

*Postage stamp graft.* A sheet of skin is cut from the donor site, cut to postage stamp size, and placed on the recipient bed. When the recipient bed is not very clean, this kind of graft permits free drainage between the grafts.

*Full cover graft.* The skin sheet is removed from the donor site and placed intact on the recipient bed. Sutures or some form of adhesive material may or may not be used to keep the graft in place.

*Lace or slit graft.* The skin sheet is removed and is run through an instrument that meshes or slits it. The meshed skin is then stretched. The edges can be sutured to keep the stretch. Exudate can be removed easily from this type of graft.

Homografts and heterografts are applied to the recipient bed in the form of split-thickness, full cover, sheet grafts. They are positioned in a vertical manner, when possible, to differentiate them from the permanent grafts, which are usually placed horizontally. They are dressed in the same manner as permanent grafts, either open or closed.

When temporary grafts are used to prepare recipient beds for grafting or to control infection, they can be changed daily or as ordered. This procedure can be done at the bedside or in a dressing room. Homograft removal may cause some bleeding. Animal heterografts usually come off very readily, with little or no bleeding. Some of the synthetic heterografts are very difficult to remove if left in place for more than a day or two. Heterografts used to dress donor areas are left in place until they fall off.

**Full-thickness grafts.** In the early stages of burn treatment, the split-

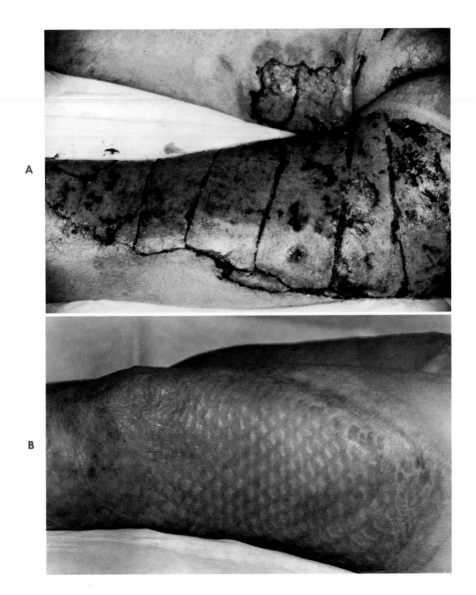

**Plate 2. A,** Healing full-cover autografts. **B,** Healed lace autograft. (**A,** Courtesy Dr. D. Ross; **B,** courtesy Dr. P. Stoddard.)

thickness graft is used most frequently. The full-thickness graft may be used early if there is a small, well-defined area of full-thickness loss that necessitates this type of graft. The full-thickness graft is used most often during the later treatment and rehabilitation phase to restore body function and cosmetic appearance. The physician tries to cover the burn wounds as soon as possible; final grafting is often delayed for a period of years. There are two main types of full-thickness graft.

*Free, full-thickness graft.* The free graft consists of the full thickness of the skin down to the subcutaneous tissue, 0.035 inch thick or more. This graft gives the best early appearance and has less late contracture. It may be used in the early stages for the well-defined full-thickness burn and for repair of burn wounds on the hands, neck and face when reconstruction is needed. It is also used to replace scar tissue and to open areas of contracture.

The free, full-thickness graft takes best on a fresh wound area. If the graft is to be used on a granulating area, the recipient bed may first be covered by a split-skin graft to determine whether or not the recipient bed is ready for take.

*Pedicle flap.* The pedicle flap consists of the full thickness of the skin and the underlying subcutaneous fat. The flap is left attached to both the recipient and donor areas until a sufficient blood supply is established to the recipient site. This type of graft is used to restore lost features and in areas where contour and bulk may be needed. It is also used in areas that may have a diminished blood supply and would therefore be incapable of sustaining a free graft. There are direct flaps (applied at the same time they are raised) and delayed flaps (raised in stages to improve their blood supply). They may also be local flaps, which are rotated to the wound from an adjacent area, or distant flaps, which are prepared at one site and brought to a distant area by stages. Flaps are used mainly in the following ways.

SLIDING GRAFT (SINGLE STAGE). Incisions are made adjacent to the defect. The skin flap is raised, rotated over the defect, and sutured to it. The donor site is then sutured closed or grafted with a split-thickness graft.

FLAP GRAFT (TWO STAGES). In the first stage, an incision is made at the donor site. The flap obtained is rotated over the defect and the donor site sutured. When the blood supply is established in the flap, the second stage is performed. In this procedure, the flap is freed from the old site and sutured in place.

PEDICLE GRAFT (THREE STAGES). In the first stage, parallel incisions are made at the donor site. A tube of skin is lifted and the area underneath is sutured. In the second stage, one end of the pedicle is freed, tailored to fit the defect, and sutured in place. After the blood supply is established, the third stage is undertaken. It consists of freeing the pedicle completely from the donor area, trimming the pedicle as needed, and suturing it in place. The immobilization required for these procedures to be successful can cause a great deal of discomfort to the patient. The nurse must make every effort to alleviate it. Particular attention must be paid to the color of the flap or pedicle. Any change must be brought to the attention of the physician.

### Preparation for split-thickness grafts

Donor sites may be shaved and cleansed prior to surgery as in an ordinary preoperative procedure. Very often the surgeon elects to prepare the donor site in the operating room.

Split-thickness grafts take best on clean, flat granulation beds. They can also take on scar tissue, if the epithelium is removed and on muscle, fascia, periosteum, and tendon sheaths. Grafts do not take well on bare bone or tendon.

In order to graft over bare bone, multiple perforations are made into the marrow cavity or the outer cortex of the bone is chipped away down to the marrow cavity. Granulating buds from the marrow cavity provide a surface for the graft. When the multiple perforation procedure is used, the process is called fenestration.

### Application techniques for split-thickness grafts

Temporary and permanent split-thickness grafts can be applied at the patient's beside, in a dressing room, or in an operating room. Sedation or local or general anesthesia can be used, depending on the physician's mode of treatment.

Some form of penicillin is usually given prior to autografting procedures. The presence of $\beta$-hemolytic streptococci on the recipient bed can destroy the graft.

The physician carefully plans the mode of coverage. For permanent grafts, priority is usually given to covering the hands and face. Areas around joints are covered before flat surfaces. Any procedure that will make the patient self-sufficient—such as arm coverage, so that the patient can feed himself, or coverage of legs, so that the patient can walk—is given priority.

When possible, the physician tries to have the donor site on the same aspect of the body as the recipient site.

### Aftercare of the split-thickness graft

One of the major roles of the nurse in the care of split-thickness grafts is to make sure that they are not dislodged. Each autograft is precious. The dislodgment of an autograft can prolong the hospital stay of the patient for several weeks. If an autograft is dislodged, it can be replaced if it is found before it dries out. It may then be necessary to wet the graft with sterile normal saline or with an antibiotic solution. Split-thickness grafts are cared for in either of two ways: they may be either left exposed or covered with dressings.

**Exposure.** Many physicians feel that grafts take better when exposed. Close observation is possible, and collections of fluid under the graft can be easily removed. If the fluid is near the edge of the graft, it can be rolled out with an applicator. If the fluid is more than 0.5 inch from the edge, it should not be rolled out. In that case, a tiny snip should be made in the tissue to allow the fluid to be rolled out without having to move the fluid a great distance.

When the exposure treatment is used, the patient must be immobilized to prevent the dislodgment of the graft. Splints, slings, or skeletal traction may be used to achieve immobilization. Flat surfaces that are grafted are easy to care for, except in the case of very young or uncooperative patients. This type of patient must be sedated and restrained for at least 96 hours.

When the perineal area is involved, the patient usually has a low-residue diet or is given paregoric to prevent bowel movements. If fecal contamination occurs, the area should be cleansed very carefully with a nonirritating soap or detergent.

**Split-thickness graft dressings.** Graft dressings vary greatly, according to the particular methods of the physician. They may be applied dry or wet.

*Dry graft dressings.* The basic dry graft dressing must be firm, with uniform compression, to hold the graft in place. The dressing must also be bulky to allow for fluid drainage away from the grafted area. The dressing should extend well above and below the grafted area. Joints should be covered to aid in immobilization. If the foreleg has been grafted, the foot should be included in the dressing. This aids immobilization and helps prevent foot drop. Splints are also often incorporated into the dressing complex to aid in immobilization.

A single layer of fairly wide mesh gauze is laid on the fresh graft. This gauze initially should be wet with a sterile normal saline solution or an antimicrobial solution to help provide better coaption of the graft to the recipient bed. A water-soluble lubricant type gauze can also be used. Heavily impregnated petrolatum gauze can cause maceration of the graft.

The inner layer of mesh gauze is secured by a single layer of stretch type roll gauze. Bulky, all-gauze dressings (24-ply or more) are used to pad the affected part. The dressing is secured firmly by stretch type bandages. If splints are used, they must be well padded and secured.

*Stent dressings.* For certain areas of the body where it is difficult to secure a dressing, a stent dressing can be used. Heavy silk sutures are placed in the normal tissue surrounding the grafted area. The ends are then tied over the dressing to hold it firmly in place.

*Wet graft dressings.* Wet dressings can be used over grafted areas. Their use is optional with sheet type grafts. Lace or slit grafts appear to have a much better take if covered by wet dressings. The solutions commonly used are silver nitrate, 0.5%, sterile normal saline, or antimicrobial agents in solution.

A single layer of mesh gauze is placed directly over the graft. This can be secured with a single layer of stretch gauze bandage. Bulky, all-gauze dressings moistened with the solution ordered are then placed on the wound.

These wet dressings may or may not be held in place by stretch type bandages; it depends on the area involved. The amount of fluid necessary to keep the dressing wet varies with the temperature of the patient and with the temperature and humidity of the environment. A dry, outer covering over the wet dressing will decrease water vaporization from the wet dressing surface. Plastic protective coverings should not be used. Too much heat can build up under the plastic and cause maceration of the graft.

### Dressing changes over split-thickness grafts

**Dry.** Dressing changes over grafted areas are done only on specific order by the physician. Usually the physician will do the initial change. If the dressing should get soiled, the initial change may be done after only a few days; if clean, the initial dressing may be left in place a week or more.

Great patience and skill are required to remove these dressings. The patient must be adequately sedated and the dressing thoroughly wet. The first look at a freshly grafted area may be discouraging, but subsequent observations may show an excellent take. That the graft is taking is indicated by its pinkish red color and its smooth adherence to the recipient bed. The area has a smooth, dry look. Areas of loss are wrinkled in appearance and may look white or quite a bit darker than the original tissue.

Subsequent dressing changes are at the discretion of the physician. Tubbing may be started as early as 2 days after grafting or may be delayed a week or more, depending on the specific order of the physician.

**Wet.** The layer of fine-mesh gauze directly over the graft and the inner bandage, if used, is left in place until the physician orders the change. The gauze pads forming the bulk of the dressing can be changed whenever necessary. If an inner bandage is not used to keep the mesh gauze directly over the graft in place, great care must be taken when changing the gauze pads not to lift up the mesh gauze. This danger is minimized by keeping the dressing well moistened.

### Aftercare of split-thickness donor sites

The donor site may be left open or covered with a single layer of dressing. Fine mesh gauze or heterografts can be used. Donor sites tend to ooze. The blood that appears forms a hard, dry crust, which serves as a good protective covering for the wound. It is essential to keep this area dry. If possible, this area should not be allowed to rest on any surface. If it does it may become "soupy" looking.

A donor site may have to be covered by a dry dressing, if it is near a recipient bed. When silver nitrate 0.5% is being used, the donor areas are also kept wet.

As the gauze or heterograft directly over the donor site lifts up, it is trimmed away and not replaced. If the donor site becomes infected, special measures may be required (see p. 126). An infected donor may need to be grafted in order to heal.

### Free, full-thickness graft dressings

Preparation of these dressings is the same as that outlined for the dry split-thickness graft dressing. Dressing changes are at the discretion of the physician but are usually done at about the fifth day. If clean, the dressings may be left in place longer.

### Care of full-thickness donor site

A small donor site may be sutured closed and treated as a surgical wound. If the donor area is covered with a split-thickness graft, it is treated in the ways previously described.

### Pedicle flap dressings

The dressing over the pedicle flap is the same as that for the free, full-thickness graft. The dressing directly over the flap should exert enough pressure to minimize venous stasis. The pedicle itself is left exposed so that it can be inspected frequently for signs of twisting or color change.

The casts and splints used to immobilize the affected parts should be well padded. The patient must be kept as comfortable as possible during the long and tedious weeks that a pedicle flap procedure may take.

Dressing changes may be done very early because of the need to check the blood supply of the flap.

### Return of function and sensation

Grafted areas are capable of sweating, secreting sebum, and growing hair. Sensory function in grafts may start about 2 months after transplantation. Touch sensation returns first, then pain and temperature sensation.

### Appearance of grafts

The physician tries to match the color of the skin taken for grafting with that of the area surrounding the burn wound, if possible. Stretching or contracting the grafted skin may change its original color. Tattooing color into grafts has been tried with some success, but special cosmetic cover makeup would seem to be the easiest solution.

An interesting fact that should be kept in mind is that full-thickness grafts can thicken or gain weight. This is especially pronounced if the patient gains a great deal of weight and if abdominal tissue has been used to cover the back of a hand.

### Treatment of scars and contractures

**Splinting.** The use of corrective splints for as long as 6 months, or until the scar tissue appears to mature, will help minimize contractures and scarring after the initial grafting period.

**Surgical treatment.** If burn scar contractures do develop during the rehabilitative period and create cosmetic and functional defects, further surgery will be needed. Scar tissue is excised, and split-thickness or full-thickness grafting is done. An operation known as Z-plasty is frequently used in the rehabilitation period to release burn scar contractures.

**REFERENCES***

*Artz, C. P., and Moncrief, J. A.: The treatment of burns, ed. 2, Philadelphia, 1969, W. B. Saunders Co.,

Brown, J. B., and McDowell, F.: Skin grafting, Philadelphia, 1949, J. B. Lippincott Co.

Cramer, L. M., McCormack, R. M., and Carroll, D. B.: Progressive partial excision and early grafting in lethal burns, Plast. Reconstr. Surg. 30:595, 1962.

Crews, E. R.: Practical manual for the treatment of burns, Springfield, Illinois, 1967, Charles C Thomas, Publisher.

Grabb, W. C., and Smith, J. W.: Plastic surgery, a concise guide to clinical practice, Boston, 1968, Little, Brown & Co.

Hartwell, S. M.: The mechanisms of healing in human wounds, Springfield, Illinois, 1955, Charles C Thomas, Publisher.

Kirov, A. A.: Restoration of the various qualities of sensation, and types of nerve endings, in free skin grafts after extensive burns, Acta Chir. Plast. (Praha) 4:240-245, 1962.

MacMillan, B. G.: The use of mesh grafting in treating burns, Surg. Clin. N. Amer. 50(6):1347-1359, 1970.

*Manteuffel, S. V., Berkich, E. J., and MacMillan, B. G.: The burn patient, management and operating room support, Somerville, New Jersey, 1969, Ethicon, Inc.

Monafo, W. W.: The treatment of burns, principles and practice, St. Louis, 1971, W. H. Green, Inc.

Sevitt, S.: Burns, pathology and therapeutic applications, London, 1957, Butterworth & Co. (Publisher) Ltd.

Shuck, J. M.: The use of homografts in burn therapy, Surg. Clin. N. Amer. 50(6):1325-1335, 1970.

*Wood-Smith, D., and Porowski, P. Nursing care of the plastic surgery patient, St. Louis, 1967, The C. V. Mosby Co.

---

*Operating room techniques are not described in this book. Those references marked with an asterisk may be used to study this aspect of burn care.

# CHAPTER 8

# Nutrition

The fluid and nutritional requirements of a burn patient depend on the age of the patient; the extent and depth of the burn injury; the presence of infection, concomitant illnesses, or injuries; and the nutritional status of the patient before injury.

## NUTRITIONAL IMBALANCE RESULTING FROM BURN TRAUMA

Metabolic disturbances and fluid imbalances are a direct result of burn trauma. Providing adequate fluids and food to meet the nutritional needs of a burn patient is one of the most important aspects of burn nursing.

### Minor and moderate burns

In minor burns, oral feedings are usually well tolerated after the initial shock of injury wears off. This may take a few hours. In moderate burns, especially in infants and elderly persons, oral feedings must be carefully monitored if given within 24 hours of injury. These patients very often are nauseated and have a tendency to vomit. Most physicians withhold oral fluids from patients with moderate and major burns for 24 hours or longer. If oral fluids are given, the patient must be carefully checked for signs of gastric dilatation.

### Major burns

In most major burns, a gastric tube is inserted to keep the stomach decompressed. Very often the gastric contents are positive for blood. The presence of blood for the first few days may be from the irritation of the gastric tube or from a transient gastritis from the effects of the burn injury. Curling's ulcer, which burn patients may develop, may appear within the first week after injury or at any time during the postinjury course.

## FLUID REPLACEMENT AND WEIGHT MONITORING

The physician is responsible for ascertaining the nature and amount of fluid given intravenously to the patient. The nurse must keep very accurate records of input and output.

Burn patients treated by intravenous fluid therapy invariably gain weight during the first few days. This gain may amount to as much as 10% of their original body weight. It is important to have the preburn weight of the patient or a weight on admission. Daily weights are indicated for the first few weeks if they can be done without unduly disturbing the patient. Weekly weighings are adequate afterward.

Burn patients can lose weight rapidly until skin coverage is achieved by healing or grafting procedures. After the patient starts diuresis (this may occur as early as the second day and continue for a week or more), a major portion of the body weight loss comes from fluid loss through the kidneys.

## FLUID LOSSES FROM THE BURN WOUND

Fluid losses through the burn areas in the form of water vapor, blister fluid, and wound exudate can be considerable. As much as 10 liters a day of water evaporation loss has been recorded by special instrumentation from a burn wound surface. The average loss of water vapor from a major burn surface is thought to be 2.5 to 4.0 liters per day.

## METABOLIC FACTORS IN FLUID LOSS

Five hundred seventy-six calories are required to cause the evaporation of 1 liter of water. The evaporation of 2.5 to 4.0 liters per day therefore causes the body to expend considerable amounts of energy to maintain thermal balance. At first the body metabolism is thought to be speeded up by the response of the adrenal glands to the shock of the burn injury. The metabolism continues to be high even after the acute period, when water vaporizational losses are diminished by the healing of the partial-thickness wounds and the covering of the full-thickness wounds with topical dressings or medications.

### Infection and fever

Infection and fever may contribute to the increased metabolic rate. While many major burn patients may have high temperatures, low temperatures are a problem in many others because the process of thermoregulation is disrupted.

### Environmental temperature

Burned patients are very sensitive to the temperature of their environment. The bodies of burn patients are exposed a great deal because of the nature of their treatments. If they are not kept free of drafts in a warm, humidity-controlled room, they shiver a great deal, thus contributing to an increased metabolism. If the patient develops a high fever, the room temperature should be lowered.

### Carbohydrate needs

Throughout the burn course high carbohydrate intake is necessary to meet the increase in body metabolism.

### Protein needs

The most significant problem in burn care, from a nutritional standpoint, is the loss of protein nitrogen associated with burn injuries. In discussing these losses, one should keep in mind that 1 gram of nitrogen represents 6.25 grams of protein. The patient soon after injury is in a state of negative nitrogen balance. There are many factors that contribute to this.

**Catabolic response.** Protein metabolism is speeded up in reaction to the initial stress of the burn injury. This catabolic response is in proportion to the extent of the injury. The catabolic phase of protein metabolism can last for many weeks. Each gram of nitrogen lost can be correlated with the loss of 30 grams of whole body tissue. Since this loss occurs through the urine, stool, and vomitus, it can be considerable: as much as 30 grams of nitrogen a day or 900 grams of body tissue.

**Exudate loss.** It has been determined that 2 to 3 grams of protein can be lost each day from each percent of body surface wound draining exudate. In some cases, loss of 7 to 8 grams was recorded.

The negative nitrogen balance contributes to the general debilitation of the patient. There is decreased muscle mass and tone, poor appetite, and increased susceptibility to infection. While healing does take place during the presence of negative nitrogen balance, it is felt to be somewhat delayed. The decrease of muscle mass is much greater than that expected from ordinary inactivity.

### Loss of fat

Large losses of fat also occur. The fat loss may average 600 grams a day in a severely burned patient. This loss may continue at a slower rate even in the presence of positive nitrogen balance.

## ORGANIZING THE FEEDING SCHEDULE

A very energetic nutritional regime, providing 50 to 80 calories per kilogram of body weight and 2 to 3 grams of protein per kilogram, is needed each day to help restore the body to equilibrium. Supplemental vitamins, especially B and C, are needed. Supplemental iron is also needed if anemia develops.

The sodium levels in the body are low at first and then rise during the diuretic and reabsorptive period. Potassium levels must be checked. In a large burn, the potassium level may rise at first and then drop sharply. Intravenous or oral supplement is needed.

When oral feedings are started, usually after bowel sounds are heard, the nurse must carefully organize the patient's feeding schedule. At first, the patient cannot tolerate large quantities of fluid or food. Small quantities, given at frequent intervals, work out much better. If feeding tubes are used, the gastric residual should be checked before each feeding. Regurgitation, with the possibility of aspiration, is an ever-present danger.

### Liquid feedings

The type of fluids given initially can vary greatly. Patients may be given Haldane's solution, which is a solution of 1 teaspoon of salt and ½ teaspoon of sodium bicarbonate in 1 quart of water; or they may be started on skim milk, whole milk, or fruit juices. One or two ounces of fluid each hour is given at first, and the amount is increased as tolerated. The patient should be encouraged to eat solid food as soon as possible.

### Solid foods

Very close cooperation with the dietary department is necessary in treating burn patients. The foods given them should be high in calories and protein. They should be foods to which the patient is accustomed. Very often the patient's family can be of great help in providing food that the patient will eat.

During the early stages of care, food may have to be served in small quantities at irregular intervals. Supplemental high-protein, high-carbohydrate liquid feedings are given, along with the solid foods, in an effort to meet the nutritional needs of the patient. This can be a vicious circle; these feedings may tend to dull the patient's appetite for solid foods, or else they give the patient diarrhea. Many commercial preparations are readily available. A blenderized formulation of the patient's regular diet should be given if possible.

## Tube feedings

When used as a major portion of the daily diet, tube feedings must provide for sufficient fluid. High protein intake leads to the production of considerable urea, and the urine must be kept diluted. The burn patient also has a high intake of milk. The immobilized burn patient can develop renal calculi very readily; sufficient fluids helps prevent this.

## PSEUDODIABETES

A high-carbohydrate, high-caloric diet can also cause a pseudodiabetes. This condition is manifested by high urine output with high urine specific gravity. The patient appears dehydrated, and hyperglycemia is present. The hematocrit, serum sodium, serum chloride, and nonprotein nitrogen level of the blood are elevated. Glycosuria without acetonuria is present. The patient is treated with insulin to control the hyperglycemia. The dehydration is corrected by giving large amounts of water by mouth or intravenously.

## MONITORING FOOD INPUT

A calorie count chart, listing all food and liquid taken by the patient, is helpful in ascertaining the patient's intake. From this a dietitian can calculate the number of calories and the amount of protein the patient takes each day. The daily totals should be checked and supplemental food added as needed.

## FACTORS HINDERING ADEQUATE NUTRITION

Pain-relieving medications, trips to the operating room, and dressing and tubbing procedures can interfere with providing proper nutrition. One must not get discouraged. Once the patient's skin is grafted and healing, the weight gain can be as rapid as the loss was.

## PARENTERAL HYPERALIMENTATION

The use of parenteral hyperalimentation to supply nutritional support for the burned patient is receiving close study in hospitals today. The use of intravenous solutions containing the necessary nutrients would seem to be the ideal answer to the nutritional needs of the patient.

There are a number of problems associated with the administration of intravenous fluids this way. While commercial solutions are available, they may need to be prepared and modified daily. This must be done under strictly aseptic conditions. Daily checks of body weight and fluid balance, fractional urine sugar concentration, blood urea, sugar, and nitrogen, and serum electrolytes are necessary checks for safe administration.

The fluid must be administered through a large vein, preferably the sub-clavian, into the superior vena cava. The danger of infection can be minimized by using strict aseptic and antiseptic techniques when inserting the intravenous catheter, when dressing the catheter insertion site, when changing the intravenous infusion tubing, or when adding to the nutrient solution.

One of the prime responsibilities of the nurse is to calculate the flow rate each hour according to the total amount of fluid ordered for the day. Because of the viscous nature of the fluid, the drip rate must be constant. The amount of fluid given each day depends on the way the body utilizes glucose. Insulin may be given with this type of feeding. If the infusion is too slow, the patient may become hypoglycemic. He may have a headache and become nauseated or listless. If attempts are made to catch up too rapidly, hyperglycemia with resulting glycosuria and osmotic diuresis can occur. The patient can become dehydrated, comatose, or convulsive. If the insulin is added directly to the infusion bottle, these problems can be minimized.

Infusion bottles should be clearly marked with time strips. Ideally, the amount given should be checked every half hour. For nutritionally de-pleted burn patients who are conscious and who have no particular gastro-intestinal disturbance, parenteral hyperalimentation disrupts the intake of normal oral feedings; the patients have no appetite. Parenteral hyperalimen-tation can be life-saving for the burn patient who is too physically depleted to get proper nutrition orally.

**REFERENCES**

Arney, G. K., Pearson, E., and Sutherland, A. B.: Burn stress pseudodiabetes, Ann. Surg. **152**:77, 1960.

Artz, C. P., and Moncrief, J. A.: The treatment of burns, Philadelphia, 1969, W. B. Saunders Co., pp. 288-303.

Cohen, S.: An investigation and fractional assessment of the evaporative water loss through normal skin and burn eschar, using a microhygrometer, Plast. Reconstr. Surg. **37**:475, 1966.

Dudrick, S. J., and others: Can intravenous feeding as the sole means of nutrition support growth in the child and restore weight loss in an adult? An affirmative answer, Ann. Surg. **169**(6):974-984, 1969.

Grant, J. N., Moir, E., and Fago, M.: Parenteral hyperalimentation, Amer. J. Nurs. **69**:2392-2395, 1969.

Harrison, H. N., and others: The relationship between energy metabolism and water loss from vaporization in severely burned patients, Surgery **56**:203, 1964.

Kukral, J. C., and Shoemaker, W. C.: The metabolic sequelae of burn trauma, Surg. Clin. N. Amer. **50**:1211-1216, 1970.

Nylen, B., and Wallenius, G.: The protein loss via exudation from burns and granulat-ing wound surfaces, Acta Chir. Scand. **122**:97-100, 1961.

CHAPTER 9

# Infection

Infection is one of the major causes of death for the burn patient. The burn patient suffers loss of skin and/or mucous membranes that provide protection for the body from organisms in the environment and in their own gastrointestinal, urinary, and oropharyngeal tracts. Necrotic wound tissue and wound exudate serve as excellent nutritive material for bacterial growth. Conditions are favorable for the development of infection.

The exact nature of the changes that occur in the systemic defenses of the body against burn injury are not known. Much research is being done in this field.

## LOCAL RESPONSE

Initially, in burn injuries, fluid accumulates in the extravascular space. Inflammatory cells in the burn tissue may fail to localize. Circulating neutrophils appear to have a diminished capacity to kill bacteria. This may be as a result of normal variations in neutrophilic function.

It is felt that, as a result of burn trauma, release of membrane-active materials cause reactive neutrophils to be trapped in the systemic capillary beds so that they cannot reach the foci of infection in the burn wound. As a result, the burn patient is very susceptible to local infection right from the time of injury.

## GRANULATION TISSUE

As granulation tissue builds up under the burn wound, increasing resistance to local bacterial invasion develops. This is caused by the ability of the granulation tissue to withdraw phagocytic cells in large numbers from the reactive capillary network. As the granulation tissue is replaced by scar tissue, this capacity appears to be lost, and the burn scar tissue becomes susceptible again to bacterial invasion.

**80**

## LOCAL CONTROL OF INFECTION

Control of bacteria in the burn wound by systemic antibiotics is ineffective, except for penicillin-type drugs, because the vasculature is injured. The drugs cannot reach the organisms in the burn wound. This focuses attention on the importance of the use of topical measures to control the wound flora. These efforts should include:

1. Removal of eschar and burn slough to minimize the quantity of necrotic material
2. Thorough wound cleansing to remove the accumulation of wound exudate
3. Use of topical agents to inhibit bacterial growth

Contamination from the physical environment should be controlled as much as possible by using aseptic wound handling technique.

## IMMUNE RESPONSES

Some of the immune responses of the body to burn injury remain intact. Recent studies demonstrate the effectiveness of the primary immune response. *Pseudomonas aeruginosa* septicemia has been prevented by the early active immunization of the burn patient with specific strains of the *Pseudomonas* organism in a polyvalent vaccine.

The adequacy of the secondary immune response can be shown by the fact that a tetanus booster injection, given after burn injury, will cause a rapid rise in the level of the antitetanus antibody, which is present in the serum. The use of hyperimmune plasma obtained from human volunteers inoculated with *Pseudomonas* resulted in only limited control of *Pseudomonas* infections in burned patients. From a practical point of view, the use of this type of therapy would be very difficult to implement on a wide scale.

Gamma globulin is synthesized and broken down rapidly by burned patients. If the circulating level of gamma globulin falls (and this is usually associated with sepsis) the amount that can be administered does not begin to meet the needs of the patient. For infants who are immunologically immature, recent trials with gamma globulin administration have shown a limited role for this therapy in combatting infection.

## BACTERIAL INFECTIONS

The organisms creating life-threatening infections have changed over the years. Years ago, *Staphylococcus* and *Streptococcus* were the major offenders. With the development of drugs to control these organisms, the gram-negative organisms (*Klebsiella, Enterobacter, Serratia, Pseudomonas, Escherichia coli,* and *Proteus*) emerged as the organisms to be feared.

At the present time, most of the gram-negative burn wound organisms can be controlled; however, gram-negative pulmonary infections, such as pneumonia, can be controlled only with the most vigorous therapy.

## FUNGAL INFECTIONS

The fungal infections are now emerging as major threats to life. Before the extensive use of topical antimicrobial therapy, around 1964, very few cases of fungal infection were reported. Since then, there has been a significant rise in that number. The burn patient seems especially prone to superimposed fungal infections. This is thought to occur as a result of the depression of cellular immunity.

Generally speaking, the inability of the burn patient to resist infection appears to be at the local level, even though there are some significant alterations of the immune mechanisms (reduced granulocytic function and initial gamma globulinemia).

## CLINICAL FINDINGS

The clinical significance of the presence of organisms on the burn wound varies with their number and species. It is the number of organisms that is the major factor. The patient's reactions to the presence and number of bacteria can be related to his general physical and nutritional condition and to the stage of burn care.

Infection causes pain, failure of skin grafts, nutritional and systemic disturbances, conversion of partial-thickness burns to full-thickness ones, and sometimes death. The higher number of deaths caused by infection reported today as compared to deaths in prior years is largely a result of the fact that more patients live through the fluid resuscitation problems of the early burn period.

Because of the nature of the burn wound, bacterial colonization cannot be avoided, but it can be minimized. Every effort must be made to reduce the number of infectious organisms in the burn wound and in the bloodstream. Sustained high-level treatments of local care, removal of eschar as soon as possible, proper supportive treatment, application of grafts, and effective topical antimicrobial therapy are all aids in reducing deaths from infection. In addition, definitive systemic therapy may be helpful, according to the type of organism involved.

## LOCAL INFECTION

Local infection implies that bacteria are present and contained within the wound. Invasive infections can be local (causing lymphangitis, regional lymphadenitis, and/or cellulitis) or they can be general (spreading metastatically to all parts of the body).

## BACTEREMIA AND SEPTICEMIA

A bacteremia sometimes occurs in a burn patient after a dressing change or tubbing procedure. There is usually a transient temperature increase. There may or may not be a positive blood culture. A septicemia usually implies persistent positive blood cultures combined with the symptoms of sepsis.

### Burn wound sepsis

The concept of burn wound sepsis should be understood because it emphasizes the importance of controlling the number of organisms in the burn wound. The phrase "burn wound sepsis" is difficult to define, but it is sometimes said to describe a wound that has more than 100,000 ($10^5$) organisms in each gram of tissue involved. The tissues surrounding the burn wound are usually involved in burn wound sepsis. The bloodstream may or may not be involved.

**Symptoms of burn wound sepsis and septicemia.** The onset of burn wound sepsis or septicemia may be acute or insidious. The symptoms may appear as early as the first 10 days after the injury, and less frequently after a month. The appearance of organisms in the bloodstream (septicemia) may be indicative of advanced sepsis or of a deep septic focus.

Many of the symptoms attributed to septicemia or burn wound sepsis (temperature variations, tachypnea, and hypotension) can also be caused by other conditions present in the burned patient.

## GRAM-NEGATIVE INFECTION

Gram-negative infection may or may not be characterized by a temperature rise and then a fall to as low as 93° F. Initially, there may be leukocytosis followed by a leukopenia. Sudden hypotension, with resultant symptoms of shock and anuria, can occur. Gastric dilatation and ileus are also usually manifested.

The wounds involved may have a bluish-black appearance with raised edges. They have a tendency to bleed very easily. Petechiae can occur in areas not burned. These patients are usually disoriented for several days until shock occurs.

## GRAM-POSITIVE INFECTION

Gram-positive infection is characterized by a spike in temperature that may reach 107° F. A leukocytosis is present. Vital functions deteriorate. The blood pressure falls, and a decrease in urine output gradually occurs.

The wounds may appear fairly dry, or they may have a purulent-looking exudate. There is dissolution of granulation tissue, and autografts and newly formed epithelium is lost. Mental confusion can be a very early symptom of impending serious gram-positive infection.

Blood cultures are not always helpful in establishing a diagnosis. One of the newer techniques is the use of quantitative analysis of biopsy specimens and of cultures from the burn wound surface. Loss of appetite, gastric dilatation, and paralytic ileus may indicate onset of gastrointestinal bleeding, but they are also frequently associated with septicemia and burn wound sepsis. The patients may also appear jaundiced.

Since the nursing staff spends considerably more time with the patient than does the physician, it is its responsibility to report all untoward symptoms as soon as possible so that the physician can institute appropriate treatment. With the onset of septicemia or impending burn wound sepsis, deterioration can be very rapid if definitive therapy is not started.

## BURN TOXINS

Dr. Martin Allgower and his associates (1971) have isolated a material from the skin of burned mice that is lethally toxic at 0.30 mg. per kilogram of body weight. It is apparently a protein with the same amino acid composition as unburned tissue, but it appears to be a polymer of the proteins of normal skin. It is antigenic and will create an antiserum when injected into rabbits. This antiserum will protect 70% of toxin-treated mice from death caused by the toxin.

The molecular weight of the antiserum is three times that of the unburned skin protein. Preliminary studies indicate that it is present in human skin as well as mouse tissue. The overall clinical significance is being studied.

### REFERENCES

Alexander, J. W.: Effect of thermal injury upon the early resistance to infection, J. Surg. Res. 8:128, 1968.

Alexander, J. W., Dionigi, R., and Meakins, J. L.: Periodic variation in the antibacterial function of human neutrophils and its relationship to sepsis, Ann. Surg. In press.

Alexander, J. W., and Fisher, M. W.: Immunological determinants of *Pseudomonas* infection in burn patients—a clinical evaluation, Arch. Surg. **102**:31-36, 1970.

Alexander, J. W., and others: Prevention of invasive *Pseudomonas* infections in burns with a new vaccine, Arch. Surg. **99**:249, 1969.

Allgower, M., and others: Everett Idris Evans Memorial Lecture—Burn toxins in mice (and men?), American Burn Association Meeting, April, 1971.

Arturson, G., and others: Changes in immunoglobulin levels in severely burned patients, Lancet **1**:546, 1969.

Artz, C. P., and Moncrief, J. A.: The treatment of burns, Philadelphia, 1969, W. B. Saunders Co.

Feller, I., and others: Use of vaccine and hyper-immune serum for protection against *Pseudomonas* septicemia, J. Trauma **4**:451, 1964.

Jackson, D. M.: Second thoughts on the burn wound, J. Trauma **9**:839-862, 1969.

Order, S. E., and Moncrief, J. A.: The burn wound, Springfield, Illinois, 1965, Charles C Thomas, Publisher.

# CHAPTER 10

# Symptoms and their causes

The course of care for the moderate and major burn patient can be quite difficult and prolonged. Many complications can occur, but these can be anticipated and sometimes avoided or minimized by prompt recognition of symptoms.

## PRIOR CONDITIONS

Many burn patients have prior physical conditions involving one or more of the body systems. Alcoholism, epilepsy, and psychologic disturbances that may have contributed to causing the burn injury can contribute to the problems encountered.

## IATROGENIC COMPLICATIONS

Many complications are iatrogenic in nature; that is, they occur as a result of the treatment used. These include drug allergies, fluid and electrolyte imbalances, urinary tract infections as a result of catheterization, septic phlebitis from infection introduced at the site of intravenous insertion, and the complications that may arise as a result of tracheostomy.

## SYMPTOMATOLOGY

Personnel involved in burn care should be aware of the possible significance of the symptoms that occur most frequently. These symptoms are best discussed according to the time period during which they occur. The symptoms commonly seen, and some of their causes, are discussed in the following sections.

### Acute phase

**Mania.** Mania can result from severe circulatory collapse, cerebral anoxia caused by pulmonary difficulty, or water intoxication. The last is caused by intracellular edema resulting from dilution of the extracellular fluid. The mania is characterized by headache, muscle twitching, blurred vision, vomiting, diarrhea, and disorientation.

**Vomiting.** Vomiting may be a sign of circulatory collapse, cerebral anoxia, acute gastric dilatation, or paralytic ileus. But sometimes it is caused by none of these and is, in fact, caused by some prior nonspecific injury.

**Disorientation.** If disorientation occurs during the first 24 hours, it may indicate a need for more intensive fluid therapy. It may also signify previous emotional imbalance, alcoholism, or drug withdrawal.

**Thirst.** Thirst may be a sign of fluid deficiency.

**Restlessness.** Restlessness is usually one of the indications that fluid therapy has not kept up with fluid loss. The patient may also be anoxic.

**Low blood pressure.** Low blood pressure indicates shock and a need for intensification of fluid therapy. It may also be caused by internal bleeding resulting from concomitant injuries.

**Sudden high pulse rate.** Sudden high pulse rate indicates shock. NOTE: Pulse and blood pressure are not as sensitive indices in burn cases as they are in cases of hemorrhage. The patient may be restless and oliguric and still have normal blood pressure and pulse.

**Oliguria.** Oliguria indicates insufficient fluid therapy, some renal damage, or shock.

**Anuria.** Anuria may indicate acute renal failure or an occluded or twisted catheter that does not allow the urine to drain properly.

**Glycosuria.** Glycosuria is usually transient and of the stress type.

**Hematuria.** Hematuria is also usually transient and is produced by the excretion of the products of broken-down red blood cells.

**Respiratory difficulty.** Respiratory difficulty may indicate pulmonary edema caused by too intensive fluid therapy, or it may indicate irritation of the respiratory tract by inhalation of noxious combustion products. Constricting eschars of chest and abdomen may also cause respiratory difficulty by interfering with the breathing mechanism.

**Poor circulation in the extremities.** Hypovolemia and shock or restricting eschars inhibiting circulation to the affected part may cause poor circulation.

## Management phase

**Restlessness or disorientation.** Restlessness or disorientation may result from fluid and electrolyte imbalances or may indicate the presence of septic conditions. Latent or overt personality disturbances may become intensified by the pain and the necessity of adjustment to the course of burn treatment. Restlessness toward the end of the management period may result from boredom or the fear of having to adjust to an outside environment. Postpubertal males are especially prone to restlessness caused by a resurgence of the libido.

**Vomiting.** Vomiting, which can occur at any time during the burn course, can be caused by gastric dilatation from air swallowing, or it may indicate Curling's ulcer, sepsis, or superior mesenteric artery compression of the duodenum. This last condition is characterized by intermittent vomiting, usually after meals. Ileus is not present.

**Loss of appetite.** Appetite lost may result from emotional reaction, pain, fatigue, unfamiliar surroundings, or unfamiliar foods. Drugs used to minimize pain may dull the appetite. Patients receiving parenteral hyperalimentation frequently have no appetite for oral feedings.

**Dysuria.** Many factors can contribute to dysuria. It can occur as a result of cystitis, which can be caused by the prolonged use of indwelling urinary catheters. Urethral strictures may also develop. Urinary catheters in place too long can cause the development of periurethral abscesses. Bladder and renal calculi may develop as the result of prolonged immobilization and infection. Cystitis or pyelonephritis may result from ascending genitourinary tract infection.

**Oliguria or anuria.** Oliguria or anuria may indicate insufficient fluid therapy; or they may be a sign of sepsis; or they can be correlated with preexisting renal disease.

**Edema.** Persistent edema may be a result of poor circulation; the patient may have cardiac decompensation. Swollen extremities may indicate the presence of thrombophlebitis. Burn patients are especially prone to the development of thrombi, which can result from hemoconcentration or from prolonged immobilization. Septic thrombophlebitis can be a result of infection caused by the contamination of the insertion sites of intravenous catheters. The affected part is tender and may have purulent drainage.

**Respiratory difficulties.** The patient may not have required incision of constricting eschars of chest or abdomen during the acute phase, but eschars can continue to constrict and may require incision during the management phase to minimize respiratory difficulties. Atelectasis, aspiration, and pneumonia are common to this period. The pneumonias are of two types: one, a rapidly confluent bronchopneumonia; the other, a metastatic form of pneumonia. This latter form is characterized by septic metastatic abscesses, which form as a result of bacterial invasion from a septic burn wound.

**Rash.** Rashes of various types are frequently seen. They may be indicative of allergic reactions to systemic or locally applied medications. In children, especially, they may indicate the presence of infectious diseases, such as measles. Heat rashes and irritations from bed linen washed in strong agents are also fairly common.

**Low hematocrit.** The hematocrit in burn patients is usually high before fluid therapy is initiated. The fall in hematocrit can be caused by red blood cell destruction, as a direct result of the thermal injury. This may be immediate or gradual, as the partially heat-injured red blood cells hemolyze. Considerable blood loss can also occur as a result of dressing and debriding procedures. Anemia can also result from a depression of the bone marrow. If *Pseudomonas* sepsis is present, hemolysins that can cause anemia are produced. A bleeding gastrointestinal ulcer, if undetected, can also cause anemia. Stools should be checked for presence of blood. Inadequate nutrition can be another contributing factor in producing anemia.

**Abdominal distention.** Ileus, which during this phase may be a result of a septic condition, frequently causes abdominal distention, as does fecal impaction. Abdominal distention may also be indicative of gastrointestinal bleeding.

**Diarrhea.** If given orally over an extended period of time, many antibiotic preparations destroy the normal intestinal flora, and diarrhea results. Highly concentrated oral or tube feedings can also cause diarrhea. Enterocolitis may develop as one of the responses to the burn injury; the exact cause of this is unknown.

**Hyperthermia.** Infection is the major cause of temperature elevations. In an extensive burn, high environmental temperature can cause the body temperature to elevate. Massive occlusive dressings or dressings enclosed in plastic material can contribute to hyperthermia. Ear infections resulting from exudate accumulation in the ear canal are frequently a cause of high temperature in children.

**Hypothermia.** Gram-negative sepsis may be indicated by hypothermia. Prolonged exposure during operating room, tubbing, or dressing procedures can also cause hypothermia.

**Loss of musculoskeletal function.** Loss of function is commonly caused by contracture. This may appear about any involved joint, but the most common sites are the neck, the axilla, the elbows, and the hands. Contractures cannot always be avoided, but they can be minimized by early skin coverage and proper positioning. The pericapsular structures beneath burned soft tissue may develop calcification in ligaments or tendons after 2 or 3 months. There is a tendency toward osteophyte formation, especially in the elbows of adults. Heterotopic, periarticular ossifications that bridge joints may form; these join the parent bone at either end and severely hamper function. Joint changes do not necessarily underlie burn wounds but can occur away from the sites of burn injury. Sepsis and prolonged immobilization are felt to be responsible for some of the functional changes that can occur in the skeletal system.

**Eye irritation.** Exudate from the burned face may run into the eyes, causing redness or infection. Fragments of singed eyelashes can also be a source of irritation. Burns about the eyes can cause eversion of the eyelids, a condition called ectropion. If the eversion is not corrected, the cornea can become dry, ulcerated, and infected. Tarsorrhaphy and early grafting can help prevent infection.

**Hypertension.** Hypertension may denote a preexisting condition in adults. In children, it appears to be associated with a significant elevation of urinary catecholamine excretion. Some encephalopathy may also be associated with hypertension. The manifestations include convulsions, irritability, restlessness or lethargy, and coma or disorientation.

**Hypotension.** Hypotension occurring in the management phase is usually indicative of internal bleeding or of a grave septic condition.

**Convulsions.** Convulsions may result from preexisting conditions (such as epilepsy) or from a head injury. Hypoxia, electrolyte imbalances, hypertension, and/or hyperthermia can lead to convulsive states. Intracranial abscess formation and meningitis related to burn wound sepsis, as well as some electrical burn injuries, may also cause convulsive disorders.

**Tissue breakdown.** In the debilitated, immobilized burn patient, decubitus ulcers are almost inevitable and difficult to prevent.

**Itching.** Itching may denote a reaction to systemic or locally applied medications. It can also result from the frequent use of hydrotherapy, since the cleansing agents used in the water sometimes create skin irritations. The healing skin has a tendency to be dry, which causes a sense of irritation.

### Rehabilitation phase

The rehabilitation phase following a burn injury may be a matter of a few months or several years, depending on the severity of the burn.

**Discharge planning.** Planning to meet the patient's needs during the rehabilitation period should be started during the initial hospitalization, well before the date of discharge. The scope of the discharge planning depends on the physician in charge and on the personnel available to implement any plans. Physical, psychologic, and social needs must all be considered.

Many adult burn victims have serious maladjustments of a physical and psychologic nature that led to the burn injury. Children suffering burn injury are often from maladjusted families.

In an ideal situation, a discharge planning conference is held. The physician, nursing personnel, physiotherapists, and social workers evaluate the needs of the patient, and plans are evolved to meet these needs. An evaluation of the family and home situation should be made before the conference.

**Nursing responsibilities.** Nursing service personnel in the hospital can help prepare the patient and the family to meet the physical needs of the patient. The patient and family can be taught in the hospital the techniques involved in cleansing, dressing, and exercising the affected parts.

**Community resources.** If the patient or family cannot handle the details of physical care, arrangements should be made by hospital personnel (nurse or public health coordinator) with the appropriate agency in the community for obtaining the necessary materials or apparatus to facilitate care. Hospital personnel should be responsible for instructing those involved with home care procedures in the techniques of burn wound handling.

**Problems of physical care.** Some of the frequently encountered problems of physical care that disturb the patient and the family in the rehabilitation stage include the following.

*Appearance of burn scar tissue.* In many instances, discoloration and rough appearance will fade and smooth out in time. This process may take several years. Certain scar tissue will have to be excised and regrafted if hypertrophy or contractures occur. Unless function is markedly impaired, surgery is delayed until tissue maturation occurs.

*Loss of function.* Loss of function caused by contractures of tissue or joint changes sometimes cannot be avoided. The patient must continue faithfully the use of splinting or positioning devices and exercise to minimize the defects, if possible. Surgery may be necessary to restore function.

*Itching.* The skin must be kept well-lubricated with a bland cream or ointment. Topical or systemic medications may be needed if there is tissue breakdown. Tranquilizers or medications that allow the patient to sleep at night are helpful. The patient should avoid the direct rays of the sun and an atmosphere that may be too dry as much as possible. Cleansing agents used in bathing must be mild and nonirritating. Clothing should be loose and of a fairly porous material to allow for exchange of air.

*Blisters.* Deep dermal burns that heal spontaneously have a tendency to blister. This condition subsides as the tissue strengthens. Many of these blisters do not open: they dry and heal readily. If the tissue breaks and the underlying tissue is exposed, the area should be cleansed and kept clean and dry. A small gauze dressing impregnated with an antimicrobial cream or water-soluble–type ointment may be necessary to protect the area.

*Unhealed wound areas.* In certain cases, the physician may decide that the patient will progress better in the home atmosphere. In some instances where open wound areas have stubbornly refused to heal while the patient is in the hospital, they may close within a matter of days once the patient is home. Careful cleansing and dressing of wounds, avoidance of mechanical trauma, and home cooking can contribute to rapid wound healing.

NOTE: A malignant ulceration that can occur in tissue that was burned is known as Marjolin's ulcer. This can occur as early as a year later, or it may have a latent period of 20 years or more. Between 1% and 2% of all skin cancers originate in burn scars. The prognosis and treatment is the same as that for other skin cancers of the squamous cell type.

*Adherent dressings.* Some wounds continue to ooze and crust for a period of time. Adherent dressings must be soaked in a cleansing solution of mild detergent or antiseptic to facilitate removal. If attempts are made to remove dressings without proper soaking, much damage can be done to the tender, viable epithelium. Daily tubbing is helpful in keeping wound surfaces clean. Occasionally a solution of equal parts of hydrogen peroxide and water may be needed to remove crusts that are especially thick and adherent.

*Continuing care.* The patient and family must be made to realize the importance of remaining under medical supervision until official discharge from care by the physician. The patient who still needs care but who does not seek it must be encouraged to return.

*Psychologic and social needs.* In addition to the many physical problems, there may be others of a psychologic or social nature. The patients may become withdrawn, depressed, and difficult to live with. Psychiatric help may be needed. Clergy and understanding friends can very often be of great help in the patient's adjustment. Social workers who can help in planning to meet the financial needs of the family can play an important role in the patient's rehabilitation. The services of a vocational rehabilitation counselor may also be needed.

**CONCLUSION**

There is no easy path for aiding the severely disfigured or functionally limited burn patient. But with proper support, he can be helped to realize his maximum capacity to lead as normal a life as possible.

**REFERENCES**

Artz, C. P., and Moncrief, J. A.: The treatment of burns, Philadelphia, 1969, W. B. Saunders Co.

Decker, R., and Nemic, B. M.: The care of patients with burns: convalescent and rehabilitation care, Nurs. Outlook 6(7):386, 1958.

Evans, E. B., and others: Prevention and correction of deformity after severe burns, Surg. Clin. N. Amer. **50**(6):1361, 1970.

Giblen, T., Pickrell, K., and Pitts, W.: Malignant degeneration in burn scars: Marjolin's ulcer, Ann. Surg. **162**:291, 1965.

Hamburg, D. A., Hamburg, B., and De Goza, S.: Adaptive problems and mechanisms in severely burned patients, Psychiatry **16**(1):1, 1953.

Harrison, H. N., and Zikria, B. A.: Management of respiratory problems in burned patients, Mod. Treat. **4**(6):1263, 1967.

Lowrey, G. H.: Sixth National Burn Seminar: Hypertension in children with burns, J. Trauma **7**:140, 1967.

Personal communications: H. Bales and M. Morrow.

Stone, N. H., and Boswick, J. A.: Profiles of burn management, Miami, 1969, Industrial Medicine Publishing Co.

# CHAPTER 11

# Special needs of the young and the old

## CONSIDERATIONS OF CARE FOR BURNED CHILDREN

### Incidence

Burn injuries rank as the third largest cause of accidental childhood deaths in the United States. Most of these accidents could have been avoided.

### Patterns of burn injury

Burn injuries of children fall into an age pattern. Below the age of 3, immersion scalds (bath water) involving the lower portion of the body are common. Spill scalds, where the toddler pulls at a coffee or a cooking pot, occur frequently. These burns usually involve part of the face and neck and one side of the arm and trunk. Flame burns are common in older children. The fluffy clothing of little girls can ignite readily from space heaters or from playing with matches. Boys tend to become involved with matches, gasoline, and bonfires.

### Evaluation of burn injury

In evaluating the depth and extent of burn injury in children, one must keep in mind that the child's skin is much thinner than that of an adult. Exposure to a heat source that would produce a partial-thickness injury in an adult may produce a full-thickness injury in a child.

When evaluating a child's burn injuries, the examiner must be alert for signs of battered child syndrome. The type of injury, location, presence of other injuries, malnutrition, or infection (denoting a delay in securing treatment) are all indications of it.

**Physiologic differences in children**

The general basic principles of burn care for adults apply to children, but there are some anatomic, physiologic, and psychologic differences that modify a child's reaction to the burn injury. The child below the age of 2 years has a relatively higher mortality rate in burns of over 20% than other age groups. Above the age of 3, the mortality patterns are essentially the same as for older groups.

**Kidneys.** The child below the age of 2 years has immature kidneys. Because of glomerulotubular immaturity, the infant kidney is unable to excrete sodium, chloride, and some other ions. It cannot reabsorb water readily, so large volumes of hypotonic urine are produced. The immature kidney cannot readily excrete large volumes of nonelectrolyte fluid; therefore, while it is very easy for an infant to become dehydrated, he also can easily become overhydrated.

**Body surface.** Infants and children have a larger body surface area in proportion to their weight than do adults. Their potential for water evaporative loss is therefore greater. This consideration affects the fluid needs of infants, and the physician will use the formulas only as a starting point. The type and amount of fluid given may need constant modification during the resuscitative period.

**Peripheral circulation.** Peripheral circulation is labile in the infant. The myocardium functions well, but the peripheral compensation is poor. Pneumonia, atelectasis, and constricting chest eschars are a real danger to the pulmonary system of the young child. While the gas and exchange ventilation is well stabilized shortly after birth, the infant's high metabolic rate, coupled with the stress of the burn trauma, leaves very little marginal reserve. The older a child is, the greater his margin of safety.

**Nursing care**

Pain-relieving medications should be kept to a minimum but not withheld. Painful treatments should be planned so that oral feedings are not interrupted. Very often a feeding tube must be kept in place to provide the necessary nutrition. The danger of aspiration is great. Gastric residuals should be checked before each feeding. The child should be positioned on the side, if possible, to minimize the possibility of aspiration.

**Monitoring.** Blood tests for serum electrolyte concentration, total protein, hematocrit, and blood gases need to be done at least every 6 hours during the acute phase. In addition to the hourly urine check for volume, pH, specific gravity, and presence of blood, urinary sodium and osmolality should also be tested.

A urine output of 10 ml. per hour for an infant under 1 year is considered adequate. Twenty milliliters per hour, should be maintained until adolescence. Thereafter, 30 to 50 ml. per hour is desirable. The urine specific gravity should be in the 1.020 range.

Pulse, respirations, central venous pressure (if needed), and temperature should be checked hourly during the acute period. The blood pressure is not always obtainable if all the extremities are involved. If the blood pressure reading can be taken it can be in a very high range (200/100). The reason for this is not fully understood. The blood pressure goes down to normal range as the child heals.

**Splinting and positioning.** Careful splinting and positioning of burned extremities and the neck are necessary to minimize contractures. Infants and children do not cooperate readily and need to be helped a great deal. If dressings or splints are in place, they must be checked carefully for proper positioning. Some children are extremely active and can inadvertently do much harm.

**Temperature control.** Burned infants and children are extremely sensitive to variations in surrounding temperature. Every effort must be made to keep body temperature within normal range. Thermal blankets, heat lamps, and an environment with temperature and humidity control are helpful.

### Complications

Burned children are as prone to the development of Curling's ulcer as adults. Ulcerative colitis can also develop. While many burn patients develop a rash of some type, in burned children there is often a rash that may be viral in origin. Children are also particularly prone to ear infections. The ears must therefore be carefully cleansed of any exudate that may accumulate.

### Psychologic support

A severely burned child needs to be observed constantly for changes in mental status as well as physical status. Physiologic factors (dehydration, overhydration, electrolyte imbalance, sepsis) may modify the child's mental status. The burn accident itself is very upsetting. Nightmares, unfamiliar people and surroundings, and painful treatments contribute to agitation. Anxious relatives may add to the general upset.

A television set, even in the very early stages of care, is most helpful. The children focus away from themselves onto something familiar. Recreational and occupational therapists can be most helpful. Schoolage children should be started on their school work as soon as possible. Kind, gentle, yet firm treatment is essential.

Whenever possible, the child should be allowed to help with treatments, such as removal of dressings, bathing, or lubrication of healed areas. Children are amazing in their ability to adjust. They must be made to feel secure and loved. An 8 year old once said to me: "How can someone who I know loves me hurt me so much?"

## CONSIDERATIONS OF CARE FOR THE AGED

Elderly persons sustaining burn injury can present many problems. Their skin is thin, like that of a child, but it does not heal the same way. The mortality rate of burns in the above-65 age group is relatively high. A burn that would be considered minor or moderate in a younger person can be major in this older age group.

### Evaluation of prior physical status

A very careful history of prior physical status must be obtained in order to minimize complications. An electrocardiogram should be done on admission. In addition to the regular laboratory tests of the blood and urine, a spinal tap should be performed if the patient's reflexes are abnormal. The patient may have suffered a stroke.

### Monitoring the vital signs

Central venous pressure lines are invaluable for monitoring the elderly. Frequent checks of all vital signs are needed.

### Nursing factors

It is very easy to overhydrate elderly patients and to overmedicate them with pain relievers or tranquilizers. While they must be kept as free from pain as possible, they must be able to be checked for their mental status.

Early mobilization, if at all possible, is essential to help prevent pulmonary complications. Elderly patients are especially prone to the development of hypostatic pneumonia. They must be turned frequently. If turning frames are used, special precautions must be taken so that the patient will not fall off the frame. Alternating pressure mattresses are helpful in preventing bed sores. Bony prominences may need special shields of foamed padding. Footboards also should be padded, since pressure sores can develop rapidly on the soles of the feet.

Fluid and nutritional needs for the elderly must be carefully planned. Feeding tubes are often necessary. As with children, aspiration can easily occur. When elderly patients are able to move about, they must be encouraged to do things for themselves as soon as possible.

**REFERENCES**

Bernstein, N. R., and Quinby, S.: Nurse adaptation to treating severely burned children, Hosp. Topics 49(6):65-69, 1971.

Bruck, H. M., Asch, M. J., and Pruitt, B. A.: Burns in children, a 10 year experience with 412 patients, J. Trauma 10:658-662, 1970.

Crews, E. R.: A practical manual for the treatment of burns, Springfield, Illinois, 1967, Charles C Thomas, Publisher.

Herrin, J. T., and Crawford, J. D.: Diagnosis and treatment; care of the critically ill child: major burns, Pediatrics 45:449-455, 1970.

Halter, J. C., and Friedman, S. B.: Etiology and management of severely burned children; psycho-social considerations, Amer. J. Dis. Child. 118:680-686, 1969.

Larson, D. L.: Shriners Burns Institute: Early care of the acutely burned child, Nebraska Med. J. 54:672-676, 733-736, 1969.

Smith, E. I., and DeWeese, M. S.: The topical therapy of burns in children, Arch. Surg. 98:462-468, 1969.

CHAPTER 12

# First aid

___

**STOPPING THE BURNING PROCESS**

The first step in giving first aid to a burn victim is to stop the burning process. The skin surface must be removed from contact with the source of heat. The heat must then be allowed to dissipate itself from the body.

**USING LIQUIDS TO DISSIPATE HEAT**

In a flame burn the patient should be made to lie flat, if possible, to minimize the inhalation of flame and smoke. Flame on clothing can be extinguished by rolling the victim on the ground or floor. Heavy coverings can also be used to smother the flames and should be removed as soon as the flames are extinguished. Any nonirritating and nonflammable liquid that is handy can also be used to put out the fire. In the home, a shower bath or immersion in a tub of cool water can be used. Outdoors, a garden hose, a swimming pool, a lake or stream, or a jug of lemonade can be used. The major point to be made is that the liquid does not have to be sterile. The ideal liquid to use is a combination of a detergent, water, and ice.

In the case of extensive burns, cold applications for removing heat from the affected tissue should only be used until the victim starts to shiver. For small burns, the cold applications can be applied until the victim is comfortable and definitive care is instituted.

**ESTABLISHING THE AIRWAY**

In the case of suspected smoke inhalation and flame and electrical burns, the airway must be checked to be sure that the victim is breathing properly. Serious respiratory problems can occur as a result of the inhalation of noxious combustion products without any signs of physical damage. The airway must be kept as clear of secretions as possible. The victim's head should be elevated. Protective coverings must not restrict chest movements.

## CHEMICAL BURNS

In the case of chemical burns, the proper neutralizing agent may not be immediately available. In that case, thorough rinsing with large amounts of water (far in excess of any normal amount) will help minimize tissue destruction. The neutralizing agents for the more commonly occurring chemical burns are as follows:

| Type of burn | Neutralizing agent |
|---|---|
| Alkali burns | Acetic acid 0.5% to 5% (1 teaspoon vinegar per pint of water) or ammonium chloride 5% |
|    Potassium hydroxide | |
|    Sodium hydroxide | |
|    Ammonium hydroxide | |
| Tear gas or mace | Sodium bicarbonate solution |
| Phosphorus | Copper sulfate soaks |

(Actually, the copper sulfate soak does not neutralize the phosphorus. It is used to give color to the phosphorus, which must be manually removed, thoroughly and painstakingly.)

| | |
|---|---|
| Acid burns | Sodium bicarbonate solution (1 teaspoon baking soda per pint of water) or sodium bicarbonate paste |
|    Hydrochloric acid | |
|    Sulfuric acid | |
|    Nitric acid | |
|    Trichloroacetic acid | |
|    Hydrofluoric acid | Sodium bicarbonate solution or paste and local injections of calcium gluconate |
| Phenol | Ethyl alcohol followed by sodium bicarbonate solution or paste |

Chemical burns can be insidious. Even after thorough cleansing, a wound that appears relatively minor at first may progress to full-thickness skin loss with destruction of underlying tissue and bone.

## ELECTRICAL INJURIES

Electricity can cause burns and burn-type tissue damage in three different ways:

1. Electrical sparks or arcs can cause an individual's clothing to ignite.

2. The heat generated by an electrical arc occurring near an individual can cause burn injuries.

3. Electrical current passing directly through the body can cause burns by the heat generated and tissue changes by the current itself. The exact effects of electrical current on tissue are not fully understood.

In injuries involving direct contact with electricity, the victim must be freed from the source of electric current as quickly as possible. Before contact with the victim, the rescuer should make sure that the current is off. The rescuer should be properly grounded and should use insulated or nonconducting materials (dry wood or dry paper will serve) to rescue the victim.

If the victim is not breathing, mouth-to-mouth resuscitation must be started immediately. Ventricular fibrillation may cause the heart to stop beating. Cardiac massage should then be used, along with the artificial respiration, until the victim can be defibrillated.

Direct contact electrical burns can be very deceiving. The external wounds may appear relatively small, but damage to underlying tissues and blood vessels can be extensive. These victims should be carefully observed for signs of shock caused by hemorrhage or intestinal perforation.

## RADIATION BURNS

Industrial radiation accidents involving thermal burns require special handling. The victim should be decontaminated at the accident site by thorough cleansing with water. Any clothing worn by the victim should be discarded. If possible, the victim should be checked at the site of the accident for the amount of radiation present in the body. The receiving facility must be notified so that radiation precautions can be set up for handling the care of the patient. One of the most important factors is ascertaining in advance the length of time that personnel involved in the care of the patient can be exposed.

## TRANSPORTATION

If the victim needs to be transported for care by ambulance or car, the affected parts need only to be wrapped in a clean, dry covering such as a sheet or towel. The foamed plastic sheeting sometimes used for emergency covering should be used with caution. It is one of the best insulating materials known. If there is still heat in the wounds, as there may be in deep thermal injuries, then the heat cannot dissipate when the plastic foam is used, and more cell damage may result.

The victim needs to be reassured. In the case of extensive, deep burns, the victim is very often not aware of the seriousness of the injury because deep burns are relatively painless. If a burn victim requires transportation to a hospital by ambulance, the driver should alert the receiving facility, if possible, regarding the nature and extent of the victim's injury.

## TREATMENT OF MINOR BURNS

For a small burn, such as occurs in the home after a very brief contact with a heat source, the treatment can be soaking or immersing the affected area in a solution of detergent, water, and ice until the part feels comfortable. A water-soluble antiseptic ointment or cream can then be applied. A clean gauze dressing can be secured. The bandage can be left in place until it becomes soiled. It can be removed by soaking the affected area in a detergent solution. A dressing may then be reapplied, if necessary.

## TREATMENT OF MODERATE OR MAJOR BURNS

In industrial clinics, hospital clinics, or a physician's office, the procedures outlined in Chapter 5 are followed.

## TREATMENT OF SUNBURN

For the treatment of extensive sunburn, immersion in a cool tub of water until the victim feels chilled is effective. A water-soluble antiseptic lubricant can then be applied. The area should be left exposed, if possible. If dressings are required, the inner layer of gauze should be lubricated with the same material so that it does not adhere.

Victims suffering from extensive sunburn may feel the effects of dehydration, nausea, vomiting, and dizziness. They need oral replacement of fluids. Fluids containing sodium should be given, such as fruit juices, cola beverages, or milk. Analgesics and antipruritic medications are also usually needed.

## TREATMENT UNDER ISOLATED CONDITIONS

If one is confronted with a severely burned victim in an isolated area where help cannot be reached, the victim must be kept as comfortable as possible with the materials at hand, following the basic principles of first aid in burn care:

1. Stop the burning process and allow the heat in the wound to dissipate.
2. Keep the victim's airway clear (the head may have to be turned to the side, to allow oral secretions to drain out).

If possible, the wounds should be cleansed and exposed to the air. The care of the burn wound may be delayed, but care must be taken not to chill the victim. If the rescuer knows that trained help will be available within a period of several hours, oral fluids should not be given to an extensively burned victim (more than 20% to 30% of the body). If the time of arrival of help cannot be anticipated, oral fluids may be started.

If conscious, the victim will be very thirsty. The ideal solution to give by mouth is called Haldane's solution. It is a solution of 1 teaspoon of salt and ½ teaspoon of sodium bicarbonate in 1 quart of water. Served cold, with a dash of lemon, it is fairly palatable. In a dire emergency, small amounts of any liquid on hand may be given: not more than an ounce or two to start, but the victim must be watched carefully to prevent vomiting and aspiration.

## LARGE-SCALE THERMAL DISASTERS

In the case of a large-scale thermal disaster, definitive care priorities should be given to victims who appear to be in the salvageable range. For adults, the disaster "rule of ninety" may be used: where the age and extent of burn add up to ninety or more, the victim has less than a 50:50 chance of survival. This rule does not apply to children under the age of 5 years. Their chances of survival are much less because they may present signs of shock with burns of less than 15%.

In planning for the care of large numbers of burn victims, a proper system of keeping records is very important. Securing the airway and administering fluids are the most important items after hemorrhage is controlled (if present) and after the burning process is stopped. The victims must also be checked for signs of internal injuries and/or fractures. Aside from the care of the eyes, if involved, and the removal of chemical agents if they are the causative agents, the actual care of the burn wound can wait, if necessary, for cleansing and definitive treatment. Available supplies must be allocated according to the salvageability of the victims. Treatment priorities are:

1. Recording history
2. Supportive care (oxygen therapy and intravenous or oral fluids)
3. Relief of pain (keep in mind that deep burns generally are not painful)
4. Prevention of infection (systemic or topical antibiotics)
5. Preservation of function
6. Care of the burn wound

**REFERENCES**

Blocker, T. G., and Blocker, V.: Simplified standardized treatment of burns under emergency conditions with particular reference to allied health personnel, Office of Technical Services, U. S. Department of Commerce, National Bureau of Standards.

Curreri, P. W., Asch, M. J., and Pruitt, B. A.: The treatment of chemical burns: specialized diagnostic, therapeutic and prognostic considerations, J. Trauma 10(8):634-642, 1970.

Gleason, M. N., and others: Clinical toxicology of commercial products—acute poisoning, ed. 3, Baltimore, 1969, The Williams & Wilkins Co.

Morton, J. H.: Disaster management of burn patients, New York J. Med. 70(12):1647-1650, 1970.

Phillips, A. W.: Burn therapy, disaster management—to treat or not to treat? Who should receive intravenous fluids? Ann. Surg. 168(1):986-996, 1968.

# CHAPTER 13

# History of burn treatment

## LOCAL CARE

The burn treatment used by Hippocrates is among the earliest on record. He recommended pork grease mixed with resin and bitumen on a warm piece of cloth to be applied as a compress on the wound. To relieve the pain of the wound, he recommended warm vinegar dressings. He also used solutions of oak bark to tan the wound.

Paulus of Aegina, a Byzantine of the seventh century, advocated the use of detergent type rinses followed by dressings containing light earths mixed with vinegar or the brine of pickled olives. Pigeon dung burned with linen and the ashes mixed with oil and applied to the wound was a favorite remedy of his.

Rhazes and Avicenna, of the ninth and tenth centuries, recommended the use of cooling agents on burns.

These early treatments may seem primitive, but on careful examination it is found that some of the same basic ingredients are used today, only in different form. The earliest treatments focused attention on the care of the burn wound and on the alleviation of pain.

The first book devoted to the care of burns was written by William Clowes in 1591. He advocated the use of grease type dressings. He also described special ointments for the treatment of burned eyes and eyelids. He advocated bleeding, as did his contemporaries. Of special interest is the fact that he left blisters intact.

Fabricus Hildanus (1560-1631) of Basel, Switzerland, wrote a book on burns in 1607. In it he describes the three different classes of burn wounds. He also described the release of contractures and the splinting of a burned hand to prevent contractures.

*Several Chirurgical Treatises* by Richard Wiseman (London, 1676) was the standard surgical work, popular in Britain late in the seventeenth century. In it Wiseman described a superficial wound as being more painful than a deep burn. He advocated the use of onion and salt beaten together as a topical dressing. This had been advocated by Ambrose Pare a century earlier. Wiseman also advised splinting to avoid contracture.

The use of carron oil was very popular in Scotland during the early eighteenth century. It was composed of equal parts of lime water and linseed oil. It was widely used until the beginning of the twentieth century.

In Edinburgh, Scotland, a brewer named David Cleghorn had many burn casualties among his factory workers. He used vinegar and chalk poultices on his patients. He did not use purges, as many of his contemporaries did. He was not inhibited by the medical men of his day. His correspondence with John Hunter concerning his treatment of burns, published in 1792, became quite famous.

John Hunter, in his book *A Treatise on the Blood, Inflammation, and Gun-shot Wounds* (1794), stressed the importance of keeping burns and scalds clean and dry. He felt that inflammation of the wounds would be minimized that way.

In 1797 Edward Kentish wrote his work *Essay on Burns*. He was opposed to the use of boiling water to draw out the "caloric" or heat, which was a popular treatment intermittently used over the centuries. He advocated the application of ice and used exposure therapy during the early stages of care and occlusive dressings in the later stages. He used oil of turpentine or alcohol as topical therapy. His recognition of the fact that a highly nourishing diet was of utmost importance was of great significance. While he purged his patients, he did not believe in blood-letting, as was still common in his day.

In 1825 a doctoral thesis of Desbarreaux-Bernard was published in Paris. It described ulcers of the stomach as a complication found in burn victims. In 1842 Curling wrote a paper on this same subject, and it was his name that became associated with the condition.

A. D. Anderson, in the *Glasgow Medical Journal* of 1828, outlined the basic principles of the burn dressing: protection, comfort, and preservation of the normal healing function. He advocated the use of a dressing complex in which the inner layer was left in place if it was not soiled. Only the outer absorbent layer was changed, thus preserving the viable healing elements. This basic dressing principle is standard practice in some dressing techniques today.

In 1815 Marjolin, whose name describes the malignant ulcer that can develop in burn wounds, advocated the use of pressure dressings. James Syme (1799-1870) of Edinburgh advocated the use of dry dressings applied with moderate firmness. He established the first burn unit in 1848; the building still stands today.

Joseph Lister (1827-1912) succeeded Syme, his father-in-law, to the Chair of Clinical Surgery at Edinburgh in 1869. The aseptic principles that he outlined form the framework for many of the basic treatments still used in burn therapy today. Interestingly enough, though, he did not apply these principles himself in his own practice. He used dressings of carbolized oil, which consisted of varying strengths of carbolic acid (2% to 16%) mixed in oil; 2% or 3% concentrations of carbolic acid are now known to cause necrosis of tissue. Some of the symptoms ascribed to his burn patients—delirium, weakness, and hypertension—might well have been the result of phenol poisoning.

Occlusive wet dressings impregnated with saline or antiseptic solutions were popular in Glasgow, Scotland, between 1885 and 1910. Doctors in Austria-Hungary before 1870 favored the exposure treatment of burns. In that year they decided to return to the use of occlusive oily or wet dressings.

One of the most prominent names in the history of burn care is that of Sneve of St. Paul, Minnesota. His article on the treatment of burns and skin grafting in the *Journal of the American Medical Association* of 1905 is a classic. He did not claim credit for the revival of the exposure treatment of burns, but he popularized it. He used salt solutions intravenously, orally, and by enema. His patients were kept clean. He also recognized the importance of pain control. His patients were kept in high-temperature rooms. His statement in 1898, "There is nothing new under the sun," still holds true for the most part today. One of the reasons that Sneve's work was of such great value was that he kept careful and accurate records.

The exposure treatment of burns is still in use today. When it is used from time to time, the use of heat is questioned. At the present time, heat lamps or heated air jets are used to help keep the wounds dry. The development of special beds, with turning devices and porous frames, have been invaluable in helping to keep the wounds dry.

The focus of burn wound care in the midnineteenth century was on the development of agents that would create a dry wound surface by tanning it or by forming a film over it. Tannic acid was used as early as 1858. It became popular in 1925, when it was advocated by Davidson of Detroit, Michigan. Tannic acid was used in different forms, extensively, until about 1944, when the hepatic necrosis found in burn victims was felt to be a result of the treatment.

Collodion and castor oil were used to create a transparent, impervious film on a burn wound in 1858 at Kings County Hospital. Paraffin wax containing naphthol, applied at a temperature of 50° to 60° C., was used widely as a burn dressing between 1918 and 1926. Naphthol can be absorbed through tissue into the system, causing renal damage, convulsive seizures, and anemia. Temperatures above 42° C. are also known, now, to cause cell damage.

Many different synthetic films made of various plastic materials have been tried without success, so far. Any film covering of "synthetic skin" must allow for transpiration of air but must minimize evaporation of water. The material must also be chemically inert and insoluble in water and tissue fluids. It must also be pliable so that the patient is comfortable.

Every conceivable substance has been used from time to time on the burn wound itself, in the form of sprays, ointments, solutions on dressings, or powders. Silver nitrate (up to 10% in strength), sulfonamides, picric acid, boric acid, zinc compounds, castor oil, acetic acid, ambrine, paraffin, chlorine (Dakin's solution), molasses, flour, alcohol, nitrofurazone, aluminum acetate, mercuric chloride, dyes (gentian violet, scarlet red, and acriflavine), silver salts (lactate and acetate), ferric chloride, colloidal ferric hydroxide, and antibiotics have all been tried. The list goes on ad infinitum.

It is interesting to note that one of the major changes in the use of a particular therapy involves a change in the concentration or strength of the material. At one time, silver nitrate 10% was a commonly used agent. At this strength it causes death of cell tissue. Today, a 0.5% solution, as advocated by Dr. Carl Moyer, is the most commonly used form.

Marfanil, a sulfonamide and forerunner of today's Sulfamylon, was used extensively in powder form during World War II. Occlusive, grease-gauze type dressings were also used, on and off, for years. In 1942 Allen and Koch popularized the use of a bulky petrolatum gauze pressure dressing.

Greasy ointments tend to macerate tissue. Topical agents today are therefore being incorporated into water-soluble ointments and creams. The medications appear to absorb faster from vehicles of this type, and wound cleansing is more easily accomplished.

A. B. Wallace, an English surgeon, revived the exposure method in 1949 for local care of the burn wound. Henry Harkins wrote *The Treatment of Burns* in 1942; this was very popular for many years. There are still less than a dozen books today dealing with the problems of total care for the burned patient, although many thousands of articles have been written on specific areas.

In 1947 the U. S. Army Surgical Research Burn Unit was established at Brooke Army Hospital in Fort Sam Houston, Texas. Colonel Edwin Pulaski helped lead this unit to the position of prominence it still holds today under the dynamic Dr. Basil Pruitt. Colonel Pulaski and Dr. Charles Tennison developed the "rule of nines" used to describe the extent of burn injury. Colonel William Amspacher helped develop the Brooke Fluid Formula. Major research programs of all kinds are being carried out in this unit today.

The organisms that cause problems in the burn wound have changed. Gram-positive organisms, such as *Staphylococcus aureus* and $\beta$-hemolytic *Streptococcus,* which were so troublesome in the past, are now fairly well controlled. Gram-negative *Pseudomonas aeruginosa* emerged in the 1960's as the great threat. Lindberg and Moncrief, working at Brooke, developed the cream Sulfamylon Hydrochloride (now used in the acetate form). This cream has proved to be effective in the control of most *Pseudomonas* infections.

The *Klebsiella, Enterobacter, Proteus, Escherichia coli,* and *Serratia* groups still pose a real threat. The topical agents used, such as gentamicin sulfate 0.1% cream, have not been officially approved for use in burn care. Fungous infections, both systemic and local, are becoming more prevalent. The use of antibiotics for topical burn wound therapy is limited by the long-term nature of burn wound care; organisms tend to develop resistant strains.

While working at Brooke, Dr. Carl Teplitz did much basic research in the early 1960's on the pathology of the burn wound. He laid the groundwork for the concept of burn wound sepsis, which focuses attention on the importance of control of bacteria in the burn wound.

The agents most widely used today are discussed in Chapter 4.

Passovant described the use of continuous water baths for burn victims in *Deutsches Archen fur Klinische Medizin* in 1858. Tub baths for burn victims were also used in Vienna in the 1880's. Friend, of Chicago, described tubbing in the *Journal of the American Medical Association* in 1895. Patients were kept in the tubs for long periods. While the patients were comfortable in the water, their infection could not be controlled.

Tubbing plays an important part in burn care today. The type of tub used, the solution in which the patient is immersed, and the length of time of immersion vary considerably. The basic goals of the procedure are the same: to keep the patient more comfortable, to afford more exercise, and to cleanse the wound to help minimize infection and to promote healing.

## SYSTEMIC CARE

In 1855 Buhl of Germany correlated burn collapse with the collapse occurring in cholera. This had been treated by Latta in 1830 and by Cantani in 1850 by sodium salts given intravenously, subcutaneously, and orally.

The nature of the changes occurring in the body fluids as a result of burn injury was described by Barceduc of Paris in 1863. He recognized the decrease in circulating blood volume and the hemoconcentration that can occur in burn victims as a probable cause of death.

Tappenheimer, of Munich, Germany, concerned himself with the study of the pathophysiology of burns in 1881. His work demonstrated the hemoconcentration that occurs in burn injury, which led to the recognition of the need for restoration of fluid volumes. He recommended the use of a transfusion of blood serum. Unfortunately, this was not available in his day. It was not until the 1930's that plasma transfusions became readily available.

Weidenfeld and von Ziembusch described their use of saline solution to save lives of severely burned patients in 1905. In the 1920's Dr. Frank P. Underhill of Yale University was a strong advocate of saline therapy. He also did extensive work on fluid losses occurring in burn trauma. His work focused attention on the importance of protein loss in burn injury.

The use of plasma and blood transfusions was not common until the late 1930's. Even with the demonstration of the protein losses and the shifts of colloid, physicians still do not agree on the use of colloid in the early stages of burn care.

Oliver Cope and Francis Moore of Boston were able to provide an explanation for the so-called hidden fluid loss in burn trauma during the early 1940's. Extensive work regarding the exact nature of these fluid losses has been done during the past 50 years. Carl Moyer did much work in this area.

In 1952 Evans of Richmond, Virginia, developed the idea of using a formula, which bears his name, to calculate fluid replacement. Colloid solutions, electrolyte solutions, and free water are all in use today. The particular fluid therapy used varies greatly. Most burned patients today survive the resuscitative period.

## GRAFTING

One of the major advances for the restoration of a burn wound victim to normal living was the development of the split-thickness autograft. In 1872 Reverdin published a paper entitled "Epidermic Graft." He used skin consisting of the epidermis and a very small portion of the dermis. The grafts were 0.3 to 0.4 sq. cm. In 1872 Thiersch modified the Reverdin graft by using larger pieces, 4 by 8 cm. He felt that these larger grafts gave better skin surface, especially over joint areas. During the period 1874 to 1876, Thiersch elaborated on the work of Ollier. The grafts they developed are referred to as Ollier-Thiersch grafts.

In 1914 Davis of Baltimore, Maryland, described a small graft that included full-thickness skin at its center. This graft, known as the "pinch graft," became very popular and was widely used until recent years. Its major drawback was the poor cosmetic appearance of the donor site and recipient areas.

Marked progress was made in the early 1920's in the improvement of the "thin skin" graft. Certain basic concepts were developed:

1. The dermis is important to the success of the graft. It provides the necessary strength and resiliency.
2. Donor site healing occurs from the epidermal appendages. Grafts can be cut as thick as possible, rather than as thin as possible, without interfering with the healing of the donor site.

These larger and thicker grafts became known as split-thickness grafts, and new instruments were developed for cutting them. In the early 1930's Blair and Brown of St. Louis developed a long, sharp, thin knife for this purpose, which became known as the Blair-Brown knife. In 1939 Dr. Padgett and Mr. Hood, an engineer, developed a drum type dermatome at the University of Kansas. There are many different types of dermatomes in use today. With them, the surgeon is able to obtain more uniform tissue and therefore better results.

The development of better techniques for split-thickness grafting has enabled the surgeon to develop larger and more uniform full-thickness grafts. Full-thickness grafts are not used extensively in the initial period of burn care. Rather, they are generally used in the rehabilitative stage, if necessary, after the condition of the patient has stabilized.

The ancient Egyptians and the Hindus of India used full-thickness grafts many hundreds of years before Christ. Their techniques were utilized by surgeons over the centuries. The first verified free, full-thickness autograft was done in Europe by Dr. Christine Bunger in 1823, using the same ancient method.

John Mason-Warren was credited in 1834 with performing the first successful full-thickness graft in America. Wolfe, of Glasgow, is given credit for introducing the full-thickness graft into clinical practice in 1875. Dr. Feodor Krause perfected the techniques in 1893 and made them more popular.

These grafts are referred to today as Wolfe-Krause grafts. Full-thickness grafts are used today in many forms.

## HOMOGRAFTS AND HETEROGRAFTS

Barionio of Italy developed in 1804 successful full-thickness grafts using a sheep as a subject. He laid the groundwork for the animal and human transplantation studies going on today. In 1816 J. C. Capue, a London surgeon, described a case in which a free skin homograft apparently survived. One must read these "successful homograft take" reports very critically. Eventually, permanent homografts may be possible. Improved methods of tissue typing may lead the way.

In 1872 Reverdin discussed the use of homografts and heterografts. At first, attempts were made to secure permanent coverage with these grafts. Today, they are used as a temporary measure until autografts are available.

Pigs, rabbits, cows, dogs, chickens, and sheep have all been used as a source of material for skin coverage. Today, pigskin, fresh or frozen, is the most widely used form of heterograft.

## THE FUTURE

The development of burn research units, such as the one at Brooke Army Hospital in San Antonio, Texas, has done much to advance progress in the burn field. Organizations such as the International Society for Burn Injuries and the American Burn Association contribute greatly to the pooling and dissemination of burn knowledge. The past few years has seen a tremendous upsurge in the interest in burn care. Burn work is no longer the orphan of the medical field.

Aided by the physiologist, biochemist, microbiologist, and statistician, the physician need no longer prescribe treatment in an entirely haphazard way. Many problems still remain. The mortality figures for burns above 60% have not changed appreciably during the recent past, but much progress has been made in the treatment of lesser burns. The future is bright.

## REFERENCES

Cockshott, W. P.: The history of the treatment of burns, Surg. Gynec. Obstet. **102**(1): 116-124, 1956.
Davis, J. S.: Plastic surgery, Philadelphia, 1919, P. Blakiston's Sons & Co., chap. 1.
Harkins, H. N.: Historical introduction, Bahama International Conference on Burns, Philadelphia, 1964, Dorrance & Co.
Lewis, S. R.: The controversy of 2,000 years—closed or open therapy? In Goldman, L., and Gardner, R. E., editors: Burns: a symposium, Springfield, Illinois, 1965, Charles C Thomas, Publisher, pp. 61-69.

Moyer, C. A., and Butcher, H. R.: Burns, shock, and plasma volume regulation, St. Louis, 1967, The C. V. Mosby Co., chaps. 5, 8, and 9.

Padgett, E. C.: Plastic and reconstructive surgery, Springfield, Illinois, 1948, Charles C Thomas, Publisher, pp. 3-89.

Shedd, D. P.: Historical landmarks in the treatment of burns, Surgery 43(6):1024-1036, 1958.

Sneve, H.: The treatment of burns and skin grafting, J.A.M.A. **45**:1-8, 1905.

Wood-Smith, D., and Porowski, P. C.: Nursing care of the plastic surgery patient, St. Louis, 1967, The C. V. Mosby Co., chap. 1.

# CHAPTER 14

# Outline summary of burn therapy

A workbook or manual outlining the details of the various treatments and the use of records should be available for all personnel giving burn care. When writing orders the physician then need only state "Sulfamylon per burn manual" or "saline wet dressings per burn manual."

The following outlines are suggested as guides for setting up work procedures. One page of the booklet should be devoted to listing the source for any special supplies needed. Example:

| | |
|---|---|
| Sterile linen | Central Supply |
| Masks, caps, and shoe covers | General Stores |
| Burn dressings | Central Supply |
|     Small all-gauze | |
|     12 × 12 all-gauze | |
|     18 × 18 all-gauze | |
|     Burn roll bandages | |

## Sample burn manual

### Contents

Introduction
Section I
    Use of the burn summary sheet
Section II
    Application of Sulfamylon Acetate cream 10%
Section III
    Application of Garamycin cream 0.1%
Section IV
    Bedside procedure for split-thickness autografts

Section V
  Care of split-thickness graft donor sites
Section VI
  Sterile wet-dressing technique for wound care
Section VII
  Care of infected donor sites
Section VIII
  Occlusive sterile dry dressing technique for burn care
Section IX
  Application of homografts (allografts) or heterografts
    (xenografts) at bedside
Section X
  Cleansing of split-thickness graft edges and suture lines
Section XI
  Care of Steinmann pin sites or K-wire sites
Section XII
  Guidelines for skin graft care
Section XIII
  Dressing for burned hand before or after grafting

I. **Use of the burn summary sheet** (see p. 47)
  A. **Purpose**
    1. To provide a concise record of vital signs in the resuscitative phase of burn treatment
    2. To provide a concise record of fluid intake and output
  B. **General instructions**
    1. The burn summary sheet is started in the Emergency Room at the time of admission.
    2. The burn summary sheet is used only until the patient is in the diuretic phase. This may begin in 2 or 3 days after injury or can be delayed for a week or more. The onset of diuresis depends on the severity of the burn injury and on the general condition of the patient. The physician should be consulted before changing to the standard intake and output sheet.
    3. The burn summary sheet is oriented for use with the graphic sheet, which is part of the regular record. The burn summary sheets covering the previous 24-hour period should be kept at the bedside at all times.

**C.  Procedure**                              **Key points**

1. Stamp patient's identification number in upper left-hand corner.

2. Record number of days post injury.

   These are important for the evaluation of the patient's condition.

3. Record daily weight.

4. Record percentage burn.

5. Chart fluid intake.

   Three basic types of fluids are used for fluid therapy. It is most important that each fluid be recorded in the proper column and the insertion site of the intravenous tube noted. The amount of fluid given in a specified time period is recorded as the numerator of a fraction. The denominator is the running total of that fluid. Fluids are usually recorded hourly. A new block is used each time fluids are changed.

6. Chart pulse rate and blood pressure.

   These vital signs are not sensitive indices of the adequacy of therapy in burns. Serious problems may exist while these signs are in normal range. However, sudden increases or drops must be reported immediately to the physician.

7. Check respiration.

   Respirations are usually elevated in major burns. The excitement of the injury, respiratory involvement, or metabolic disturbances can cause this. The patient must be checked carefully for signs of pulmonary edema.

8. Check central venous pressure (CVP).

   CVP monitoring is helpful in infants, elderly people, and patients with history of cardiac and renal disease. Readings must be taken at the same level each time. Ascertain from physician the point at which a change in reading should be reported.

9. Check urine output.

The urine output is a very important guide in ascertaining patient's condition. It is one of the most important guides in determining the state of the patient's hydration. The intravenous fluids are adjusted according to the amount of urine produced and the specific gravity of the urine. The physician determines in advance the point at which a change in urine output is reported. Too much urine production in the early stages can be as serious as too little urine. An output of 30 to 50 ml. per hour is the acceptable adult average, and 10 to 35 ml. per hour is the average for a child (varies with age). The urine should be checked for blood, pH, and specific gravity.

10. Check use of nasogastric tube.

Most moderate and major burns need nasogastric tubes as a matter of routine. Gastric dilatation and vomiting can occur with even a minor burn. Any medication or fluid given by nasogastric tube (as well as orally) must be carefully measured and recorded.

11. Check for emesis.

If the patient has emesis, type, volume, and manner of vomiting must be recorded and reported to physician. The emesis should be checked for blood. If the emesis is small in amount and at first seems to roll out from the mouth, do not be misled. This may be overflow from a severely dilated stomach.

12. Check stool.

Stool should be checked for blood. Ulcers in the gastrointestinal tract can develop very early in a burn patient.

13. Remarks.

Record special medications or symptoms.

**II. Application of Sulfamylon Acetate cream 10%**

  **A. Purpose**

    1. To keep bacterial reproduction to a minimum

    2. To help prevent partial-thickness wounds from converting to full-thickness wounds because of infection

    3. To help prevent burn wound sepsis (bacterial invasion of unburned tissue under and around the burn wound)

  **B. Equipment needed**

    1. Sulfamylon Acetate cream 10%

    2. Sterile gloves

    3. Sterile scissors

    4. Thumb forceps

    5. Nonadherent absorbent pads

    6. Fine-mesh gauze

    7. Gauze squares

    8. Stretch gauze bandage

State source of supply.

  **C. Procedure**

**Key points**

1. Give pain medication as ordered at least 20 minutes before starting procedure.

Sulfamylon Acetate may cause stinging, especially on areas of partial-thickness wounds.

2. Cleanse wounds thoroughly using the method appropriate for that patient.

  a. Tub in physiotherapy

  b. Tub in stationary tub using nonirritating cleansing agent

  c. Shower

  d. Cleanse wound at bedside with warm, clean, or sterile water and nonirritating cleansing agent. Rinse thoroughly with clean or sterile water or saline.

3. Place nonadherent absorbent pad under areas where cream is to be applied.

Paddings contacting burn wounds must be nonadherent. They must hold the cream against the wound but must be thick enough to allow the wound exudate to be absorbed away from the wound surface.

4. Debride loose tissue from the wound.

Any tissue hanging free that can be cut from the burn wound without causing bleeding should be removed using scissors and forceps.

5. Apply Sulfamylon cream to burn wound using a gloved hand. The cream should be applied so that the burn wound is not visible (2 to 4 mm.).

Deep burn wounds invariably become infected. They are avascular in nature. Systemically administered antimicrobial medications cannot penetrate the burn wound. Topically applied medications must be used in sufficient quantity to be effective.

6. Use new glove each time re-entry into Sulfamylon jar is necessary.     OR

7. If Sulfamylon cream slides off certain areas, the cream may be buttered on to strips of single-layer fine-mesh gauze or single-layer gauze squares and placed on wound. Secure with single-layer stretch bandage.

The burn wound may have so much exudate that the cream just slides off. Gauze holding cream in place should be no more than two layers thick.

8. Replace Sulfamylon cream on wound any time it comes off.

9. Keep pads underneath burn wounds clean. If the padding sticks, sterile saline or sterile water may be used to facilitate removal.

In burns over 50%, check with physician.

10. Observe patient for reaction to Sulfamylon. Before reapplying check for rash and observe respirations. NOTE: Sulfamylon is usually applied twice a day.

Some patients may develop an allergy to the cream. Acidosis may develop and manifest itself by tachypnea or hyperpnea.

### III.   Application of Garamycin cream 0.1%
   A.   **Purpose**
      1.   To keep bacterial reproduction to a minimum
      2.   To help prevent partial-thickness wounds from converting to full-thickness wounds because of infection
      3.   To help prevent burn wound sepsis (bacterial invasion of unburned tissue under and around the burn wound)
   B.   **Equipment needed**
      1.   Garamycin cream 0.1%
      2.   Sterile gloves
      3.   Sterile scissors
      4.   Sterile thumb forceps
      5.   Nonadherent absorbent pads
      6.   Fine-mesh gauze strips or squares
      7.   Stretch gauze bandage
   C.   **Procedure**

**Key points**

1.   Give pain medication as ordered at least 20 minutes before starting procedure.

Cleansing of the wound before application of the cream may be painful.

2.   Cleanse wounds thoroughly, using the method appropriate for that patient.

   a.   Tub in physiotherapy
   b.   Tub in stationary tub using nonirritating cleansing agent
   c.   Shower
   d.   Cleanse wound at bedside with warm, clean, or sterile water and nonirritating cleansing agent. Rinse thoroughly with clean or sterile water or saline.

3.   Place nonadherent absorbent pads under areas where cream is to be applied.

Paddings that contact burn wounds must be nonadherent. They must hold the cream against the wound but must be thick enough to allow the wound exudate to be absorbed away from the wound surface.

4.   Debride loose tissue from the wound.

Any tissue hanging free that can be cut from the burn wound without causing bleeding should be removed using scissors and forceps.

5. Apply Garamycin cream as follows:

   a. Directly to burn wound, using a gloved hand.  OR
   b. Using fine-mesh strips or single-layer squares of gauze that have been buttered with the cream. Secure with stretch type gauze.

Garamycin application should be painless with no stinging or burning.

The cream spreads easily and quickly becomes invisible. Therefore, care must be taken to ensure that entire area is covered.

This method is used for wounds having considerable exudate, since the cream may slide or be rubbed off if directly applied. Avoid overlapping the fine-mesh gauze.

6. Replace Garamycin cream as ordered.
7. Keep pads underneath burn wounds clean. If the padding sticks, sterile water or saline may be used to facilitate removal.
8. Observe patient for reactions.

Wounds are usually cleansed and cream reapplied twice a day.

Garamycin can be nephrotoxic and can cause auditory or vestibular ototoxicity. Urine should be monitored. Report dizziness or vomiting immediately to the physician.

IV. **Bedside procedure for split-thickness autograft**
   A. **Purpose:** A split-thickness autograft affords permanent coverage of denuded surface with skin obtained from patient's own body. This coverage affords protection from infection and helps prevent evaporative water loss. It also helps restore the affected part to function and improves appearance.
   B. **Equipment for skin preparation**      **Key points**

Utility cart on which are placed:
   1. Skin prep tray (disposable)

      Set up outer wrapping as sterile field.

   2. Cleansing agent
   3. Sterile water or sterile normal saline

      Use for rinsing.

   4. Razor

      Shave donor site and area around recipient site before prep is started.

5. Sterile Kelly clamps (two)
6. Small sterile dry sponges
   
   Number varies according to size of area.
7. Sterile plastic surgery debriding set (forceps and curved Mayo scissors)
   
   Recipient area might need further debriding before procedure is started. Obtain sets from Central Supply.
8. Sterile gloves
   **C. Equipment for grafting procedure**

**Key points**

Utility cart on which are placed:
1. Suture set containing forceps and scissors
2. Appropriate sutures    Check with physician.
3. Appropriate dermatome    Check with physician. Obtain from Operating Room.
4. Sterile towel on which are placed:
   a. Kelly clamp
   b. Prep basin containing 2 × 2 sponges moistened with tincture of iodine (mild, 2%)
   c. Prep basin containing 2× 2 sponges moistened with Isopropyl alcohol, 70%
   d. Prep basin containing sterile normal saline solution
   e. 10-ml. syringe
   f. No. 25 needle
   g. Two No. 26 needles
   h. Donor site and graft dressing material, if ordered
   i. 3 × 4 sponges
   j. Knife blade
   k. Knife handle
   l. Sterile mineral oil, 2 oz.
5. Two masks
6. Sterile gloves (2 pairs)
7. Procaine hydrochloride    Check strength and type wanted.

8. Alcohol sponge
9. Four sterile towels
10. Treatment blanket
11. Waste disposal container

**D. Procedure**

**Key points**

1. Explain procedure to patient. Position him comfortably, with donor and recipient areas exposed.
2. Drape patient with draw sheet.
3. Place folded treatment blanket over patient's chest in such a way that procedure cannot be viewed by the patient.
4. Assist the physician as follows:
   a. Open gloves.

   Once gloved, the physician will maintain sterile technique, so nurse must assist by handling the nonsterile items.

   b. Open prep tray and remove after use.
   c. Open procedure tray.
   d. Prep diaphragm of procaine hydrochloride bottle with alcohol sponge and hold bottle while physician fills syringe.
   e. Open dermatome set and place on sterile field.
   f. Assist as necessary in helping patient maintain correct position.
5. Observe patient for untoward reactions.
6. Leave area exposed as physician orders.

   Donor site requires drying; grafted areas require positioning away from drying light.

7. Discard disposables, rinse reusables, and leave on sink in utility room.

8. Remove knife blade from der-matome and discard blade in "sharps bucket." Return der-matome to Operating Room.
9. Record in nurse's note the pa-tient's reaction, the location of the two sites, and the care given them (exposed, immobilized, other).
10. Check graft periodically if ex-posed; if fluid has collected under tissue, gently roll fluid out using a sterile swab.

It may be necessary to use sterile scissors to nick the blister.

V. **Care of split-thickness graft donor sites**

A. **General discussion:** The epidermis and part of the dermis, vary-ing in thickness from 0.008 to 0.020 inch, have been removed. The donor site is therefore a partial-thickness loss wound and must be protected from infection and mechanical trauma or it will convert to a full-thickness wound requiring grafting.

| B. Procedure | Key points |
|---|---|
| 1. Ascertain location of donor sites and grafted areas. | Grafted areas are sometimes cov-ered. Dressings are left in place. If possible, donor areas are left ex-posed. |
| 2. Gently remove pressure dress-ings over donor sites as ordered by physician. If inner layer of fine-mesh gauze or heterograft has been used, leave in place. | Physician will remove pressure dressing himself or leave specific order for removal, usually after 6 hours for a child or after 12 hours for an adult. |
| 3. Position patient *so that donor area does not contact any sur-face.* | Extremities may have to be sus-pended or propped up. A bed cradle with lamp may be needed to keep bed clothing off body. |
| 4. Expose donor site to heat light for 15 minutes every 2 hours, or as ordered. | Dry donor sites heal more rap-idly. If grafts are near donor site, they must at the same time be pro-tected from drying too rapidly. |
| 5. Tub patient as ordered by phy-sician. | Cleanliness is important for rapid healing. |

6. Trim fine-mesh gauze or hetero-graft, as it separates from donor site. *Do not* replace fine-mesh gauze or heterograft unless specifically ordered.

7. Lubricate donor area after all fine-mesh gauze or heterograft is removed and area is healed. NOTE: Heterografts, animal or synthetic, used on clean donor areas become very adherent. They are left in place until they come off spontaneously.

Use appropriate lubricant as ordered. Healing takes place in about 10 days. Well-cared-for donor sites can be used many times.

VI. **Sterile wet-dressing technique for wound care**
   A. **Purpose**
      1. To help soften the crusts of partial-thickness wounds
      2. To soften the eschar of full-thickness wounds
      3. To help prepare granulation beds for grafting
      4. To protect grafts
   B. **General discussion:** The solution to be used for the wet dressing and the frequency of change of dressing are generally specified by the doctor. Dressings that become soiled between ordered changes should be brought to the attention of the physician in charge. As a general rule, complete changes are ordered at least twice a day. In the case of wet dressings over grafts, the inner layer of gauze, if used, *is not changed* unless there is a specific order from the doctor. Wet dressings must be kept well moistened at all times.

   C. **Equipment needed**

**Key points**

1. Two sterile basins of appropriate size.

State source of supply.

2. Sterile gloves (2 pairs)
3. Plastic bag for soiled dressings
4. Protective towels

Use to protect the bed under the patient.

5. Dressings of appropriate size ($18 \times 18$, $12 \times 12$, or small compress)

Order size according to area involved.

6. Fine-mesh gauze

7. Plastic debriding set
8. Asepto syringe
9. Appropriate solution

Apply sterile normal saline or solution as ordered (Sulfamylon, silver nitrate, silver acetate, others).

10. Stretch gauze rolls

**D. Procedure**

**Key points**

1. Medicate patient with analgesic, as ordered, if necessary.
2. Remove soiled dressings.

Do not remove inner layer of gauze over grafts unless specifically ordered by the doctor.

3. Cleanse unburned areas.
4. Apply fine-mesh gauze, if ordered.
5. Apply appropriately sized gauze dressings.

Fill sterile basin with appropriate solution and immerse dressings for complete saturation.

6. Secure dressing with stretch type bandage.
7. Cover wet dressing with a dry blanket or towel and change when it gets damp.

If patient is very hyperthermic, the dry cover should not be used until the patient's temperature is down. *Do not enclose wet dressings with plastic.*

**VII. Care of infected donor sites**

   **A. General discussion:** Continuous wet soaks are needed until the wound exudate appears clean. At this point, donor area can be exposed to light and air. Wound will not epithelialize properly if infection is present. If the donor area has been converted by infection to full-thickness loss, the area will need split-thickness grafting. Wet soaks, properly used, help produce a clean flat granulation bed for receiving the graft.

   **B. Equipment needed**

   **Key points**

1. Fine-mesh gauze strips

Used only if original fine-mesh gauze on donor site has been removed.

2. Sterile all-gauze dressings
3. Dry cover of appropriate size

4. Soak solution, as ordered by physician
5. Sterile Asepto syringe

   **C. Procedure**

   **Key points**

1. Apply single layer of fine-mesh gauze strips over donor area if original gauze has been removed. Do not overlap.

   This assists in debriding necrotic material and in keeping wound surface smooth.

2. Apply all-gauze dressing of appropriate size.

   These dressings should be thick enough to keep moisture in and to allow for absorption of infected material away from wound surface.

3. Wet the dressing with the solution ordered.

4. Use appropriately sized dry cover.

   Change as often as necessary.

5. Change complete dressing as ordered.

   Dressing should be changed at least four times a day. Rewetting a soiled dressing reinfects wound surface. Original fine-mesh gauze that is adherent is not removed unless it lifts up easily from wound surface.

**VIII. Occlusive sterile dry dressing technique for burn care**

    **A. Purpose**

        1. To afford protection to burn wound
        2. To hold topical agents against wound surface
        3. To keep wound surface dry
        4. To help preserve position of function of affected parts

    **B. General discussion:** Occlusive dry dressings as used in burn care are usually a dressing complex. An inner layer of gauze material of a fine-mesh type is placed next to the wound. This layer varies according to the stage of wound care. For debriding purposes the inner layer should be dry, with the mesh of the fine-mesh gauze of a fairly wide type. A water-soluble lubricant on the inner layer of gauze is used over healing wounds and grafted areas. This gauze must be permeable to allow for flow of exudate away from the wound surface. The mesh should not be wide enough to entrap epithelial buds. The next layer of dressing material must be fluffy and bulky to afford protection and to hold the exudate away from the wound surface. The dressing complex is best held in place by stretch type bandage. The complete dressing must be firm but not constricting.

**C.  Equipment needed**

1.  Sterile normal saline

2.  Four sterile basins of appropriate size

3.  Appropriate cleansing and rinsing solutions
4.  Sterile gloves (2 pairs)
5.  Plastic bag for soiled dressings
6.  Appropriate protection for use under areas being dressed
7.  Appropriate inner fine-mesh gauze
8.  Appropriate topical agent, if ordered
9.  All-gauze bulk dressings
10.  Stretch bandages
11.  Forceps and scissors (two of each)
12.  Swabs

**D.  Procedure**

1.  Medicate patient with analgesic, as ordered, if necessary.
2.  Remove soiled dressings.

Key points

Use for soaking dressings, to facilitate their removal, if necessary.

Use for cleansing and rinsing the burn wound and unburned areas, if patient is not tubbed or showered before procedure.

Sulfamylon, Garamycin, silver sulfadiazine, Polysporin.

Use for debriding, if necessary.

Use for milking exudate from grafts.

Key points

Do not remove inner layer of fine-mesh gauze over grafts unless specifically ordered to do so by physician. Patient may be put in tub to facilitate removal of dressings, if ordered, or dressings can be soaked with appropriate solution before removal.

3. Cleanse wounds in appropriate fashion.

Tubbing, shower, or bedside cleansing may be done with appropriate cleansing solutions.

4. Debride any necrotic tissue as needed, or remove fluid accumulations under grafts.

5. Apply appropriate inner dressing (dry gauze for debriding, lubricated gauze over healing areas and grafts).

Lubricant can be Furacin or antimicrobial cream, as ordered.

6. Apply appropriately sized all-gauze bulk dressings.

7. Secure with stretch-gauze bandages.

Bandages must be secure but not constrictive.

NOTE: Massive occlusive dry dressings are rarely used during the early care of burn wounds. Their major use today is for dressing hands or individual limbs. They may be necessary to protect grafted areas.

IX. **Application of homografts (allografts) or heterografts (xenografts) at bedside**

A. **General discussion:** Homografts or heterografts can be easily applied or removed at bedside, when they are used as biologic dressings for short periods of time (1 to 4 days). Grafts used in this fashion help clean up infected areas, test for receptivity of an autograft, and stimulate epithelialization in partial-thickness wounds. The patients are generally more comfortable when their wounds are covered.

B. **Equipment for preparation of the recipient bed**

**Key points**

Utility cart on which are placed:

1. Skin prep tray

Set up outer wrapping as sterile field.

2. Cleansing agent

3. Sterile water or sterile normal saline

Use for rinsing.

4. Razor

Area around recipient site should be shaved before prep is started.

5. Sterile Kelly clamps (two)

6. Sterile dry, small sponges

Quantity depends on size of involved area.

7. Sterile plastic surgery debriding set (curved Mayo forceps and scissors)

Recipient area may need further debriding.

8. Sterile gloves
9. Sterile towels

Use for protection of bed linen.

### C. Equipment for grafting procedure

**Key points**

Utility cart on which are placed:
1. Sterile towel

Use for laying out graft tissue prior to application.

2. Sterile scissors and forceps

Use for trimming grafts to size.

3. Sterile cotton applicators

Use to smooth down grafts.

4. Appropriate dressings, if used

See Dry or Wet Dressing Procedure.

5. Sterile gloves

### D. Procedure

**Key points**

1. Explain procedure to patient and position comfortably, with recipient area exposed.

Procedure is not painful unless extensive cleansing and debriding were done prior to graft application.

2. Medicate with appropriate analgesic if necessary, as ordered.
3. Cleanse recipient area.

If possible, patient should be tubbed or showered before procedure is started.

4. Open containers holding grafts. Place grafts on sterile surface.
5. Cut grafts to appropriate size and apply to recipient bed.

Be sure cut side is facing down.

6. Smooth grafts in place.

Restrain and position patient so that grafts are not dislodged.

7. Cover with dressing, if ordered.

Grafts may be left exposed or dressed.

8. Record date and site of graft application.

9. Check grafts periodically, if uncovered.

If fluid has collected under the tissue near the edge of the graft, roll the fluid out gently. If fluid has collected near the center of the graft, nick the raised area and express the fluid gently.

NOTE: If homografts or heterografts are left in place for no more than 3 days, they can usually be easily removed during tubbing or at bedside by the nurse. If left in place longer, they may become very adherent and have to be removed by the physician. Heterografts on donor sites are left in place until they fall off spontaneously.

X. **Cleansing of split-thickness graft edges and suture lines**
   A. **Purpose:** To minimize crust formation, which retards healing
   B. **General instruction:** Initiate this procedure as soon as crusts appear along a suture line between grafts or at the edge of a graft

   C. **Equipment needed**

   **Key points**

   1. Sterile toothpick type applicators

   Number according to size of area to be treated.

   2. Sterile basin containing a 1:1 solution of hydrogen peroxide and sterile water

   Use for mixing the peroxide solution.

   3. Sterile scissors and pickup forceps
   4. Strips of fine-mesh gauze
   5. Antimicrobial cream

   D. **Procedure**

   **Key points**

   1. Apply hydrogen peroxide solution along suture lines or graft edges, using sterile applicators.

   Allow several minutes for crusts to be thoroughly softened. Several applications may be necessary.

   2. Gently remove crusts using dry sterile applicators or forceps.
   3. If ordered, apply antimicrobial cream along suture lines or on open areas between grafts.
   4. Cut fine-mesh gauze pieces to cover open areas between grafts.

   Fine-mesh gauze protects the granulation bed and minimizes hypertrophy. *Do not allow gauze to overlap onto grafted area.*

## XI. Care of Steinmann pin sites or K-wire sites
A. **Purpose:** Skeletal traction aids in the positioning of the patient undergoing extensive grafting procedures. Wound care is greatly facilitated. Concomitant fracture injuries, if present, can be corrected, and contracture deformities can be minimized.
B. **General instructions:** If the legs of a patient are in traction, the head should be above the level of the heart.
C. **Equipment needed**
  1. Small sterile basin
  2. Sterile applicators
  3. Hydrogen peroxide
  4. Sterile normal saline
  5. Antimicrobial cream or ointment or antiseptic solution
  6. Sterile 2 × 2 compresses

D. **Procedure**

1. Inspect pin sites daily.

**Key points**

If clean and dry, no action is necessary.

2. If drainage is present:
  a. Using sterile applicators, clean areas around pin sites with a 1:1 solution of hydrogen peroxide and sterile normal saline.
  b. Apply appropriate cream, ointment, or antiseptic solution around pin site, if ordered, using sterile applicator.
  c. Place 2 × 2 gauze around pin site, if ordered by physician.
  d. Cleanse infected pin sites every 6 hours and as needed.
  e. Report any signs of infection or movement of the pin.
  f. Consult physician regarding any shifting, increasing, or decreasing of weights.
  g. Be sure weights are hanging free.

h. Release weights when changing linen or transporting patient.

i. Check hands or feet of involved extremities for dropped position.

j. After pins are removed, pin sites must be cleansed until healed.

NOTE: If wires are used to aid in positioning, the care of the skin around the wires is the same as that used with the Steinmann pin.

**XII. General guidelines for skin graft care**

1. Obtain the cooperation of the patient by explanation of procedure.

2. Adequately sedate patient.

3. Position patient in as comfortable a manner as possible.

4. Change dressings only on specific order by physician in charge.

5. Observe grafts frequently for dislodgment, signs of infection, and color change.

6. Because heat lamps may be used to dry the donor site, protect exposed split-thickness grafts from excessive drying out by shielding if the graft is located near the donor site.

7. Make sure that initial postgraft tubbing is no more than 10 minutes. Tubbing is done only on specific order by physician in charge.

8. Do not let exposed grafts and donor sites come in contact with any surface. If absolutely necessary, as with circumferential wounds, then they should rest on surfaces padded with smooth-surfaced absorbent pads that can be easily removed without tearing the tender epithelium.

9. Keep healed grafts and donor sites well lubricated.

10. Protect legs that have been grafted by light, stretch type gauze bandage and heavy stretch support bandages before patient is allowed to ambulate. Remove support bandages when patient is in bed.

11. If possible, tub patient prior to grafting procedure.

12. If patient has been on reverse precautions and sterile linen, discontinue these only *after the final permanent grafting procedure.*

### XIII.  Dressing for burned hand before or after grafting
  A.  **Purpose**
1.  To hold position of function and to minimize contractures
2.  To keep antimicrobial creams on wound surface
3.  To protect grafted areas
4.  To keep wound surface clean

NOTE: Hand dressings on grafted areas are changed only when specifically ordered by physician. Hand dressings on patients being tubbed twice a day are usually *done once a day* after the morning bath.

  B.  **Equipment needed**                 **Key points**

1.  Sterile gloves
2.  Fine-mesh gauze strips (dry or water-soluble cream gauze)

Use as ordered by physician. Water-soluble cream gauze is used over grafts or burn areas. Dry fine mesh can be buttered with antimicrobial cream or used plain for debriding purposes.

3.  Small all-gauze compresses

These are available from Central Supply 25 per bag. The number used depends on the size of areas involved.

4.  Gauze sponges, 2 × 2
5.  Kling rolls

These are available in 4, 5, or 6 inches. Ascertain number and size according to need.

6.  Plaster (for initial dressing)        Ascertain type and size needed.
7.  Webril                                Use for lining splint.
8.  Appropriate size basin with hot water   Use in making plaster splint.

9.  Barrier towels

Use under areas to be dressed and in sterile field for preparing dressing materials.

  C.  **Procedure**                        **Key points**

1.  Cleanse hand and forearm in appropriate manner.
2.  Wrap each finger individually with single-layer fine-mesh gauze.

Physician will specify type to be used. Fingertips are left exposed.

3. Dress dorsal and palmar hand surface and forearm with appropriate single-layer fine-mesh gauze.
4. Open one small all-gauze dressing completely. Place in palm of hand.
5. Separate fingers with 2 × 2 gauze sponges.

   Gauze must be well tucked into web space. Skin surfaces should not touch.

6. Secure fine-mesh gauze and gauze sponges with Kling.
7. Pad arm with all-gauze dressings.

   Padding should be bulky enough to protect but must allow for proper positioning of splint. This allows metacarpal phalangeal joint to fall into flexion. (Patient should be able to hold a tennis ball.) Wrist should be dorsiflexed about 25 degrees. Splint, after it is used the first time, should be protected from soiling. Stockinette covered with a clear plastic should be used.

8. Place plaster splint in position. Distal end of splint is placed at proximal crease of palm.
9. Secure plaster splint with Kling. Be sure thumb is in position of abduction with some opposition.

   Dressings must be secure but must not constrict.

NOTE: See Fig. 5-3.

# Index

**136**